I0464453

Master Tung's Acupuncture Primer

by Robert Chu, PhD, L.Ac., QME

Revision 1.1

ITARA Publications

飲水思源

Master Tung Ching-chang

董公景昌先生

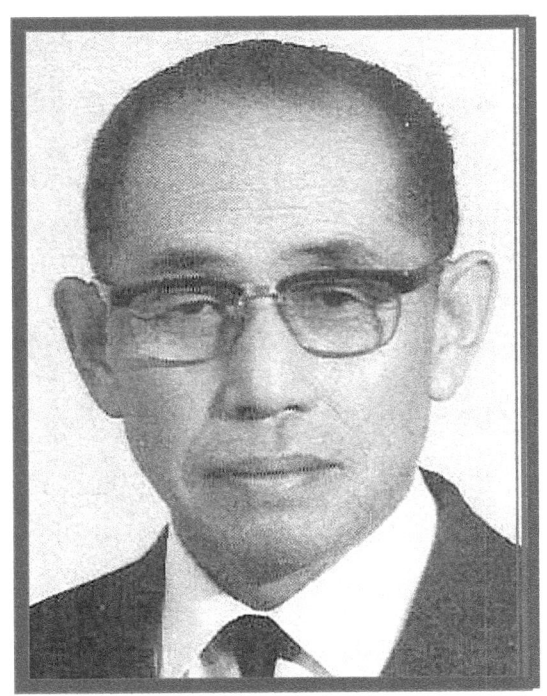

May 23, 1916 – November 7, 1975

Disclaimer

Please note that the author and publisher of this book are NOT RESPONSIBLE in any manner whatsoever for any injury that may result from practicing the techniques and/or following the instructions given within. Since the material deals with prior knowledge of acupuncture described herein, it will be too complex in nature for some readers to engage in safely, and it is essential that a licensed acupuncturist be consulted prior to application.

Dedication

To Pauline, Simone, Sean, Leo – my family.

To my students, apprentices, interns and colleagues around the world, thank you for your inspiration and journey.

NOTE ON ABBREVIATIONS USED IN THIS TEXT

In this text we use the following abbreviations for the various channels:

Lu = Lung Channel

LI = Large Intestine Channel

St = Stomach Channel

Sp = Spleen Channel

H = Heart Channel

SI = Small Intestine Channel

UB = Urinary Bladder Channel

K = Kidney Channel

Pc = Pericardium Channel

SJ = Sanjiao Channel

GB = Gallbladder Channel

Liv = Liver Channel

Ren = Ren Channel

Du = Du Channel

Table of Contents

AUTHOR'S PREFACE

Many will wonder why I wrote another book to introduce Master Tung's Acupuncture. After all, I have already written three other books on the clinical basics with **The Best of Master Tung's Acupuncture**, **Master Tung's Acupuncture for Pain**, and **Master Tung's Acupuncture for Internal Medicine Disorders**. This book is a **Primer** – an introduction of the quintessential basics. Something that a person who has not attended my seminars could read in a couple of hours, and immediately familiarize themselves with the core concepts, imaging, channel methods, and a few "go-to" points, and immediately apply the magic of Master Tung's Acupuncture in the clinic. It is not exhaustive in theory, details, or intricacies, but shows the power of the system to a TCM trained acupuncturist and immediately benefit by it. Those that wish for more can then delve into my works and the works of others to get a more complete picture.

When I first started working with Master Tung's Acupuncture in acupuncture school, I read the available books of that time and wished there was a simple book to present the information. Since the average acupuncturist already is familiar with over 400 points, *why scrap that and begin another system*? But in the way I wrote this Primer, they can simply add to the information they have and then immediately apply this in the clinic.

In this book, I introduce what I consider the quintessential principles, concepts, and points of Master Tung's Acupuncture. There are many books on Master Tung's Acupuncture which introduce all of the 740 Tung family points. I would certainly recommend Dr. Wang Chuan-min's book, **An Introduction to Tung's Acupuncture,** or Dr. Young Wei-chieh's **Lectures on Tung's Acupuncture - Points Study**, but often these books may be too much for the beginner and do not let the beginner grasp useful concepts or how to use Master Tung's Acupuncture immediately and effectively. For beginners and intermediate students of Tung's Acupuncture, I wrote the books **The Best of Master Tung's Acupuncture, Master Tung's Acupuncture for Pain**, and **Master Tung's Acupuncture for Internal Medicine Disorders**. This book is geared for the absolute beginner to give them an idea of what Tung's Acupuncture is for. But don't underestimate the power of the content of this book. It will certainly transform your practice.

Most acupuncturists simply add the Tung points to their already memorized TCM Acupuncture point prescriptions, and as a result, make a mess out of their acupuncture. They do not have a simple and elegant rationale for using the system. But the idea in this book is to use the powerful 14 Channel system you are already familiar with and make use of the Master Tung system immediately.

The idea is to use the channels to treat and identify disease, somewhat counter to the way that TCM acupuncturists are trained

today. Most TCM trained acupuncturists are taught to memorize
formulas and prescriptions according to some sort of *Zang Fu*
diagnosis, Eight Pattern diagnosis, or Five Element diagnosis. They
are just taught to memorize lists without thinking about the logic of
the way acupuncture was originally designed.

The methods in this book are of my own paradigm. I draw from
Master Tung's Acupuncture and also draw from Classical
Acupuncture, that is, Acupuncture from the classics, prior to the
1950's committee based acupuncture that was born in China, which
was using herbal based diagnosis. This is the method that I have
used for over a decade to teach in the *International Tung's Acupuncture
Research Association,* or **ITARA** for short.

In my opinion, one only needs about a hundred points in the clinic,
but one finds more than one way to apply them. The idea is to
choose the handful of points that you will use for the disorders you
see in the clinic. But this is personal to everyone's clinic, as the cases
you see will be different than mine.

I dislike overly drawn out discussions on theory, but prefer that
application be one's guide, so I keep to essential discussion briefly. I
also dislike secrecy, so I hold back no "alleged" secrets from anyone
who wants to learn the real art. The feudal master-disciple
relationship still exists in Tung's Acupuncture, along with dogma and
secrecy. My goal is to provide clinical education, to help end suffering

in the world, and help English speaking acupuncturists improve their proficiency through the vehicle of Master Tung's Acupuncture.

Many get overwhelmed when they refer to other media on Master Tung's Acupuncture. The existing numbering system is poor and nonsensical, the names of the points are all in Chinese, and the English translations of the names are poorly selected, and even worse, point locations are off. Some have deliberately tried to differentiate Master Tung's Acupuncture and regular acupuncture by stating that it is "non-channel acupuncture" - nothing could be further from the truth!

Also, little is done to approach the body of work on Master Tung's Acupuncture in a practical manner, and for one to use clinically on a daily basis. It is hoped that the reader can use these few points here and achieve amazing results in his or her practice, as these are the same points I use in my own practice daily with amazing results!

In Chinese, we always speak the phrase of *Yin Shui Si Yuan* 飲水思源 – that is to remember the source of the water we drink. In the case of Master Tung's Acupuncture, we must always remember and give credit to *Tung Ching-chang (Dong Jing Chang,* in *pinyin),* who shared his family legacy with the world. He not only shared his family secrets, but also his own genius in recreating his system through memory and experimentation. There is no doubt that part of his art was of his own innovation. It is a shame many acupuncturists today do not give credit where credit is due and have even claimed Master Tung's teachings *as their own creation.*

I would like to thank Dr. Young Wei-chieh, for his instruction in this method that he learned from Master Tung. I thoroughly applied the theoretical teachings Dr. Young taught me in the clinic to prove them to myself, my students, my apprentices, and my interns, as well as, my patients. What I present here certainly works and is reasoned out using solid acupuncture principles. I also studied meticulously the written works of other Tung practitioners and discussed with other practitioners and experimented with their methods in the clinic for over a decade and saw and recorded great results.

I would also like to thank Dr. Wang Chuan-min, who has come out recently to teach his version of the Classical Master Tung System. His version, complete with the Five *Zang* Channels of the Tung family, is a unique preservation of the Tung Acupuncture system. Dr. Wang generously shared with me original texts and corrections he made of Master Tung's early works in Taiwan, and answered all of my questions regarding Master Tung.

I would like to acknowledge Esther Su, the premiere disciple of Miriam Lee, and renowned master of Tung's Acupuncture, for her generous help. I am touched by her openness and generosity for sharing with me her personal notes and early teachings of the late Miriam Lee, the true pioneer of Master Tung's Acupuncture in the USA.

I would also like to acknowledge the late Dr. Richard Tan (Tan Te-fu) for his pioneering efforts in the USA and internationally. His charisma and teaching certainly opened up the world of Master Tung's Acupuncture through his Balance Method, a compiled method combining the works of my late Master, Chen Chao, creator of *I Ching Ping Heng* (Balance) Acupuncture, Master Tung's work, Dr. Lee Kuo-chen's work, Dr. Young Wei-chieh's work, Dr. Fang Yun Peng's work, and many others, although with some innovation on his part. I was not an apprentice of Dr. Tan, but certainly enjoyed his numerous lectures, and could see where he got his sourced information from, as we drank from the same well of knowledge.

As no work gets done without assistance, I would also like to thank Robert Ting, for his artwork.; Jack Chang, L.Ac., for proofing the work and discussing ideas with; and Trish Lowe for her assistance on several illustrations. Also a special thanks to Bob Wong, L.Ac., of Melbourne, Australia for his cover photo on Ling Gu and Da Bai, two of Master Tung's best known points, and his *Art of Acupuncture*. Thank you all for your invaluable help!

Using this book in the clinic

In this book are indispensable, everyday points for using Master Tung's Acupuncture, as well as how I approach using the fourteen channels acupuncture with Tung's Acupuncture. As I have said in my previous works, Master Tung's Acupuncture needs to be simple, practical, effective, should be painless, easily accessible and have powerful results immediately.

Master Tung taught in three phases during his life in Taiwan, after 1949. When Master Tung first came to Taiwan, he used regular acupuncture points, but used them according to channel relationships and circuits. These are what are presented here in this book. One would not have to learn any Tung family system points, as this would already have made you a superior acupuncturist.

During that time in Taiwan, other acupuncturists began to mimic him and get similar results, so he started using his family set of 740 points. Since the war, the Tung Family notes and books were destroyed, so Master Tung had to recreate the understandings of his system through memory and experimentation. This is the period in which he accepted disciples to share in the Tung Acupuncture legacy. And this is the most common teachings reflect this period of development.

Toward the later phase of his life, his last five years of so, he freely combined regular acupuncture points and Tung family points.

I try to share with all of my students the three phases and try to make them see the advantages of each. Obviously, the last phase of his life where he freely combined Tung's points with classical points, shows an even greater flexibility, but one must have a strong basis in both the 14 Channel system of acupuncture and Tung's family points.

All is laid out here, with no secrecy and made simple. I am a firm believer that basics are already advanced, and what we call "advanced" is often just the basics applied. All the tools needed for the first and third phase are in this book. The complexity is putting it all together and applying it in the clinic with great results.

For those looking to have quick clinical results without trying to master the Tung system, or for treating pain in the acupuncture clinic, as well as Internal Medicine disorders, should refer to my two other works, *Master Tung's Acupuncture for Internal Medicine* and *Master Tung's Acupuncture for Pain.*

Many incorrectly think that Master Tung's Acupuncture is just a great acupuncture system *for treating pain conditions,* but in reality, its applications are broad and *can treat all types of diseases.* To pigeon hole Master Tung's Acupuncture as a system only good for pain is self-limiting.

Essentials

Acupuncture is a targeting system. What is necessary is that the acupuncturist first identify the involved channels. After this, they need to use the imaging or holographic system, insert needles and retain them for a half hour. Treatment frequency is two to three times a week, for at least one course of treatment consisting of ten visits. After the initial course of treatment, the patient may be re-evaluated and additional courses of treatment may be suggested, if necessary. Of course, if you are an herbalist, you may prescribe herbal formulas as homework. In my clinic, I generally prescribe herbals, but with discuss this in a forthcoming text.

Acupuncturists, in addition to their needling, need to cultivate their *Yi Nian* (意念) – their focus and intention in needling the target. If they are lacking in this often non-discussed subject, they often do not get clinical results. An acupuncturist should have a clear understanding of why each point was selected, and for the purpose of each needle. While needling, the mind is in a calm, unhurried manner, as if in meditation or *Samadhi*. In my opinion, many of today's acupuncturists lack this training, and simply use memorized prescriptions and "spray and pray". What is needed is seated meditation, breath work, *Qigong* or yoga practices, mantra recitation, and standing meditation.

Although, Master Tung's Acupuncture consists of 740 family points in all, plus unique applications of the 14 channel points, it is not important to use them all. In my experience, 20 – 30 points are all one needs in general daily clinical practice. In this book, I give you 20 – 30 Tung family points, but you easily combine them with the points you learned for licensure, so you can handle most clinical situations.

One could also say that a working knowledge of a 100 or so, points is all one would ever need. Many enthusiastic students try to learn all 740 points in a four day course and find that they can't apply them in the clinic, or with limited success. I always remind my students that less is more. They should concentrate on things that are immediately useful for them in the clinic. That is the reason why I wrote this book, and have taught seminars all over the world.

In my teaching of Master Tung's Acupuncture, I always choose points that are *painless, easily accessible, and have powerful immediate results,* so I do not focus on a lot of thigh points, finger points, or prick a lot. Patients in the United States do not like painful acupuncture, nor do they like to disrobe, or have patience to see results. Since society has become increasingly litigious, I also avoid any malpractice issues. So this is my rationale for my particular style of Master Tung's Acupuncture system.

Some like to needle the finger points as they are quite powerful and have immediate result, but the drawback is that since the hands are well innervated, the patients may howl in pain. It may be fine for a free clinic overseas where you are doing charitable treatments to develop your practice, but certainly for not paying patients.

In needling for pain disorders, we needle the contralateral, or opposite side. The *Huang Di Nei Jing Su Wen's Miu Ci* chapter and the *Ling Shu's* chapter on the *9 needles, 12 Yuan Source suggest to needle the opposite side.* For example, in the Ling Shu, we are advised:

"Diseases in the upper, use the lower region points;
Diseases in the lower, use the head;
Diseases in the right, use the left;
Diseases in the left, use the right."

- A Complete Translation of The Yellow Emperor's Classics of Internal Medicine and the Difficult Classic – Henry Lu Translation

However, if pain is bilateral, we *may* choose to needle bilaterally, but often, I find this wasteful and redundant, and may actually blunt the effect of needling. In the event of bilateral pain, I borrow from classical acupuncture, where needling is applied on the left for men, and right for women. This eliminates the need for needling bilaterally.

In my clinical experience, it matters very little which side you actually needle, as the human body is one organism and always strives for balance and homeostasis. Also, my making a statement of the importance of intention and focus is again reiterated. One simply cannot hit a target if they are not focused on it.

In Tung's acupuncture, points on limbs, ears, head, and face treat general disorders and are generally treated with fine needles. By fine needles, I mean to use very thin needles with a guide tube. Generally, I use a standard 36 or 38 gauge needle, as I have the thinness and control in needling. Many of my Tung Acupuncture contemporaries are heavy handed and do strong *De Qi* sensation while needling, manipulate the needle and use thick gauge needles. I repeatedly demonstrate the effectiveness of my *painless* method in all my classes.

Needling is applied with a simple guide tube and disposable needles and retained for about a half hour clinically. Of course, one should observe proper needle angle with straight or diagonal insertion necessary when needling the torso or over vital areas. In my opinion, one does not have to manipulate the needle with Tung's Acupuncture.

Needling depth is standard as in TCM acupuncture. In Tung's Acupuncture, as expounded Young Wei-chieh, we observe the

Five Tissues needling. These draw from Classical Acupuncture. For example, in *Ling Shu* Chapter 9, we are advised:

"For bone, use bone…

for tendon, use tendon…"

- A Complete Translation of The Yellow Emperor's Classics of Internal Medicine and the Difficult Classic – Henry Lu Translation

In *Su Wen* Chapter 55, we are taught:

"Insert into the tendons to treat the tendons;

Insert into the muscles to treat the muscles."

- A Complete Translation of The Yellow Emperor's Classics of Internal Medicine and the Difficult Classic – Henry Lu Translation

This would explain that relationship of needling into the tissues and the depth of our needling. From deductive reasoning, we certainly understand that needling shallowly would affect the skin, and pricking into the blood vessels will affect the vessels.

The classics have a wealth of experience in sharing with us the wisdom of the Ancients. In terms of depth and retention, the *Ling Shu* Chapter 38 suggests:

"For a fat person, (use) deep and long retention;

For a thick, dark person, deep and long retention;

For a thin person, shallow and quick retention;

For average person, use a normal amount of time and depth;

For a tough person, more needles, frequent treatment, and deep and long retention;

For infants, shallow and quick retention, twice a day."

– A Complete Translation of The Yellow Emperor's Classics of Internal Medicine and the Difficult Classic – Henry Lu Translation

This is deep information. Let's start with analyzing an average person. We are advised to "use a normal amount of time and depth". This means we should retain the needles for clinically about 30 minutes, and insert to about 0.5 cun in depth.

So naturally, we are advised for the heavier set or the strong, ("a thick, dark person person, probably a Southern Chinese, who probably did manual labor), (use) deep and long retention; that would be deeper than the 0.5 cun depth and longer than 30 minutes.

For the skinny and frail, and this would include the elderly, we are advised to do "shallow and quick retention". This would be less than the 0.5 cun needling depth, and shorter than 30 minutes duration.

For those who do pediatric acupuncture, the *Ling Shu* advises us to do "shallow and quick retention, twice a day." This means no retention of needles, as babies do not stop moving or squirming. But it suggests to increase the frequency of needling to twice a day.

This leads us to dosage of a course of treatment. Many clients ignorant of acupuncture are astounded when I tell them I need to see them two to three times a week, for a total of ten sessions to administer one course of treatment. Of course, In China or Taiwan, this would be completely acceptable. But overseas, patients may scoff at coming in to the clinic so frequently.

Of course, I tell them that al medicine needs a proper dosage. And I use an example. Let's say you woke up with a headache and took two tablets of Acetaminophen, and eight hours later, you have a headache again. You don't say, "Darn pills! They don't work!" because when you look at the label, you see that the proper dosage according to Drugs.com, "Adults and adolescents weighing 50 kg and over: 1000 mg every 6 hours or 650 mg every 4 hours, with a maximum single dose of 1000 mg, a minimum dosing interval of 4 hours, and a maximum daily dose of acetaminophen of 4000 mg per day." (Of course, they should go see the acupuncturist instead of taking Acetaminophen...)

If we look to the *Ling Shu* again, we are given the advice:

"For chronic disease, give treatment every other day"

So for acupuncturists only seeing a patient once a week, they are not giving a proper dosage of acupuncture.

It would be good for modern acupuncturists to heed the wisdom of our ancestors and make an inquiry into the classics.

Master Tung's Numbering system

Master Tung's Acupuncture attempted to establish a numbering system in various books in Chinese, but it is easier to memorize the Chinese names, as they relate to the function of that point.

The numbering system is poorly conceived and theoretically distributed amongst 12 portions of the body. They have no relevance clinically.

Personally, I do not use the numbering system at all, as the system is rather meaningless, but just allows one to cross reference points amongst the many authors of Tung's acupuncture.

None of the Tung Acupuncture teachers I know ever use the numbering system in conversation or teaching, perhaps recently, only by those who cannot pronounce the Chinese names of the points. Often I get requests of students of mine telling me about their success with using 77.01, 77.02 and have to do what all have to do – I have to look them up.

Since I ask all of my students to just memorize twenty or thirty points and know them well, I feel Chinese and non-Chinese native speakers can learn them, as they are often also schooled in Herbalism and the Romanized *Pin Yin* system.

The 12 portions of the body include:

11 – finger points

22- hand points

33- forearm points

44 – upper arm points

55 – Sole of Foot points

66 – Top and Side of foot points

77- Lower Leg points

88 – Thigh points

99 – Ear points

1010 – Face and Scalp points

DT – Dorsal Torso points

VT – Ventral Torso points

Another category of **A** points is Master Tung's Appendix points. These are points added after the standard numbering system was implemented.

Also, my own personal points, and points of others who work within the Tung Acupuncture system may not have numbers, only names.

In my opinion, this entire system needs revamping or should be scrapped.

Finger Lines

Each digit of the hand is divided into 8 lines. Dr. Young in his book, **Dong Shi Qi Xue Zhen Jiu Xue**, Zhi Yuan Publishing, Taiwan 1992, named the palmar side lines as named A through E, I named the lines F – H, on the dorsal side, following his example. This helps in locating the points on the fingers:

Line A is the radial side of the finger, at the junction of the red and white skin

Line B is the bisecting line between Line A and Line C

Line C is the palmar centerline of that particular finger

Line D is the bisecting line between Line C and Line E

Line E is the ulnar side of the finger, at the junction of the red and white skin

Line F is the bisecting line between Line E and Line G

Line G is the dorsal centerline of the finger

Line H is the bisecting line between Line G and Line A

Please refer to the diagram below:

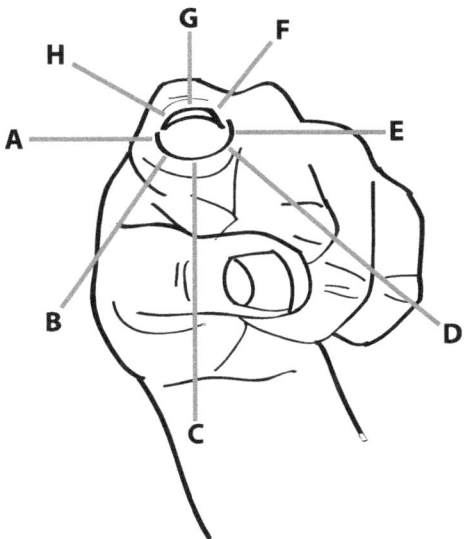

Proportional measurement between the epicondyles of fingers

Also, it is important that we use proportional measurement between the epicondyles of the segments of the phalanges. This is illustrated below:

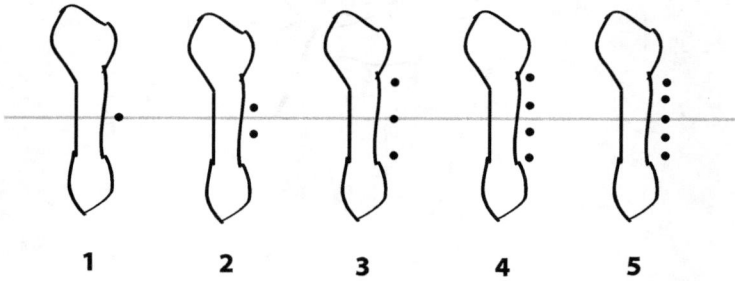

Healthy Channels of the Twelve Organs

The Twelve Channels include the Lungs, Large Intestine, Stomach, Spleen, Heart, Small Intestine, Urinary Bladder, Kidney, Pericardium, San Jiao, Gall Bladder, and Liver. These are not exactly the same as the Western Medicine in function, and may or may not pertain to the Western medical organ. By knowing the basic functions of each organ and channel, we can understand what the normal healthy body looks like. Once you know what a healthy body looks like, it's easy to diagnose the unhealthy body. We will be sharing here what these basic functions are.

It is assumed here that the majority of my readers are already Licensed Acupuncturists and already are familiar with the Channel system, pathways, and individual points.

There is a passage from the *Ling Shu*, Chapter 10, in which Le Gong is asking the now proficient Huang Di for instruction on the Channels:

Le Gong said: I want to know all about meridians (channels) at once.

Huangdi answered: A doctor should know the theory of meridians (Channels) in order to know the condition; prognosis of all kind of diseases, and how to regulate excess or deficiency of diseases.

- Ling Shu Acupuncture English edition Hardcover, 2007 Published by Ling Shu Press, ISBN 0-9770605-1-9, Copyright No: TX 6-601-362

In Classical Acupuncture, the channels are the diagnosis, and the treatment of all diseases. Regulating the channels for excess and deficiency is the key.

One time, I had tea with Dr. Young, I asked him a question, "What is the secret to acupuncture in treating diseases?"

Dr. Young's reply, "Once you can identify the involved channels, you can treat any disease."

Another time, I had tea with the world famous Dr. Chao Chen, my master in I Ching Balance Acupuncture, and I asked him in similar vein, "What is most important to know in acupuncture?"

Of course, I assumed Dr. Chen would speak about the I Ching, yin yang, Ba Gua, the sixty four gua, seasons, and other things deriving from the I Ching (aka Yi Jing) …

Dr. Chen's response was startling, "Robert, when you know the channels, you're more than halfway there!"

This lesson resonated throughout my early studies in acupuncture, which had me pursue from all disciplines Chinese, Korean, French, English, Japanese, American, Vietnamese, in which I was insatiable, and my pursuit to know, was all encompassing.

Of course, tackling the classics were my only source of condolence. I studied the classics, such as the *Jia Yi Jing*, *Nan Jing*, *Zhen Jiu Da Cheng*, and the *Ling Shu* – these were the keys to lost knowledge. In fact, the compiler of the *Zhen Jiu Da Cheng* (The Great Compendium of Acupuncture and Moxibustion), Yang Ji Zhou advised, "Better to forgo the points than the channels".

The TCM classics of *Chinese Acupuncture and Moxibustion*, Shanghai Text, and *Fundamentals of Chinese Acupuncture*, were a product of a new, herbal committee led acupuncture.

Quite basically, we should view the healthy channels as:

Lungs – The Lungs control respiration, and disperses into the skin and hair.

Large Intestine – The Large Intestine receives waste and absorbs water

Stomach – Receives and "decomposes" food

Spleen – Transforms and transports food into blood and energy, controls the flow of blood in vessels, and dominates the muscles and functions of the four limbs, opens into the mouth, and manifests in the lips.

Heart – Is referred to as the "Emperor", and dominates blood and vessels, houses the Shen (Spirit), and opens into the tongue

Small Intestine- Receives food, aids in digestion, and absorbs water and nutrients.

Urinary Bladder – Stores and releases urine

Kidney – Stores Jing (Essence) and governs growth and maturation and reproduction, dominates water metabolism, assists in gathering of Qi from the Lungs, dominates the bone, builds marrow, and brain, manifests in hair, opens into the ears, controls the orfices of urination and bowel movement

Pericardium - protects the Heart

San Jiao – Acts as a passageway for Qi and its functions, assists all the other organs in their functions

Gall Bladder – Stores and excretes bile, governs decision making

Liver – Stores and purifies blood, maintains the free flow of Qi in the body, controls the tendons and the nails. The Liver also opens into the eyes.

Pathogenic Channels

Often, I joke that in our profession that we should not be called "Acupuncturists", but rather "Channelpuncturists". I state this because we rely on the channel signs and symptoms, rather than the points or other methods of diagnosis. As long as we needle the channel, we can get an effect. If one point doesn't show an effect, we should insert a second needle. If severe, we should add a third needle into the channel. We should see an immediate effect if treating for pain, or at least a cessation of certain symptoms the patient is suffering from internal or chronic cases. We then retain the needles for a period of one half hour. Describing this method is showing the Master Tung *Hui Ma Zhen* method in application.

If there is no immediate effect, we must have diagnosed incorrectly, or the patient is on certain medications, requires surgery, or some other remedy.

We are here reminded of pathogenic channel signs and symptoms:

Ren Channel Symptoms
Hernia, leukorrhagia, and masses and lumps in the abdomen. Since the Ren Channel is considered the Sea of Yin, it may be used in the treatment of all Yin disorders. Other signs and symptoms may include pregnancy and fetal nourishment problems, irregular menstruation, spontaneous abortion, and infertility.

Ren Channel

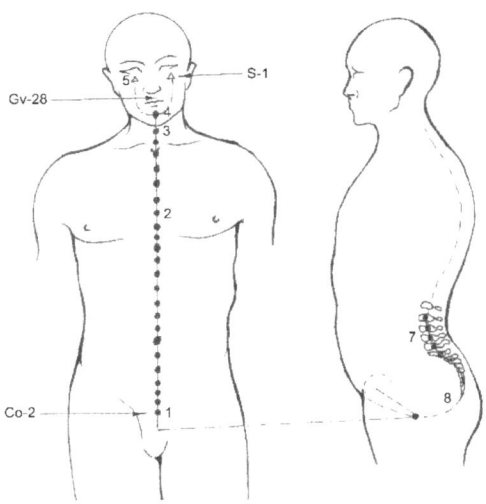

Du Channel Symptoms

Pain and stiffness in the spinal column, and opisthotonos. Since the Du Channel is considered to be the Sea of Yang, it may be selected and used in all Yang disorders. Other signs and symptoms may include pain of the back, mental disorders, infantile convulsion.

Du Channel

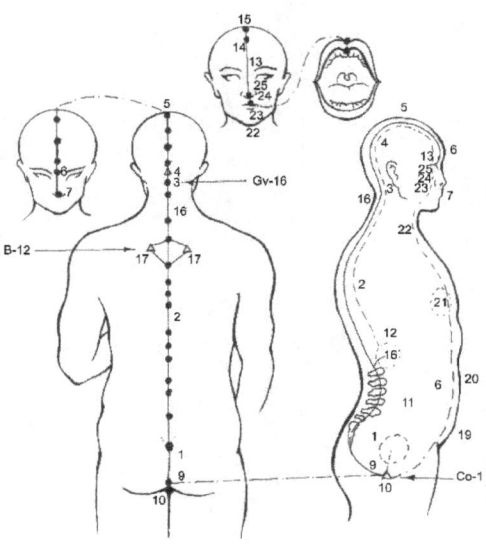

Lung Channel Symptoms

Cough, asthma, shortness of breath, hemoptysis, common cold, fullness in the chest, sore throat, and other disorders (e.g. pain) along the course of the channel. Also used for grief, sadness, melancholy. Other signs and symptoms may include fever and aversion to cold (with or without sweating), nasal congestion, headache, pain in the supraclavicular fossa, chest, shoulders, back, cold pain along the channel on the arm, wheezing, and dyspnea, rapid breathing, oppression in the chest, expectoration of phlegm, dry throat, abnormal urine color, restlessness, spitting of blood, heat in the palms, fullness and distention in the abdomen, thin stool diarrhea, frequent urination, yawning, urinary incontinence, cramping and pain along the course of the Lu sinew channel that if severe results in accumulation lumps below the ribs, qi counter flow, tension along the ribs. The Lung Channel is most active on the Xin day.

Lung Channel

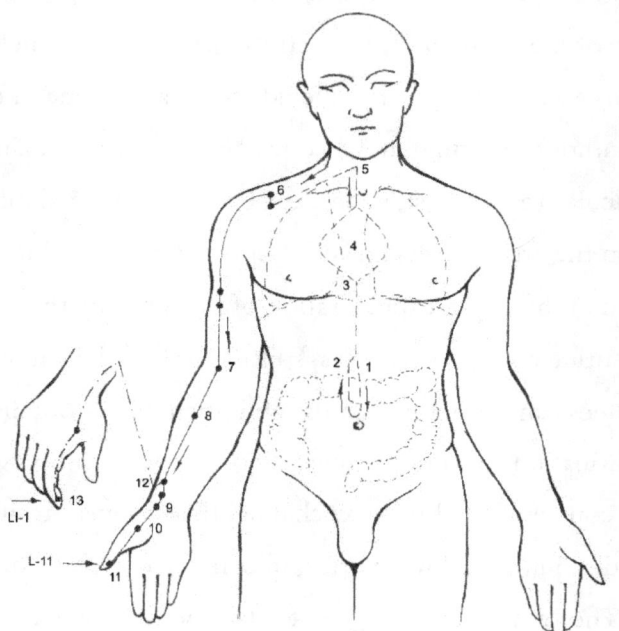

Large Intestine Channel Symptoms

Abdominal pain, borborygmus, diarrhea, constipation, dysentery, toothache, sore throat, stuffy nose, and the other disorders (e.g. pain) along the course of the channel. Also used for grief, sadness, melancholy. Other signs and symptoms may include fever, parched, dry mouth with thirst, nosebleed, toothache, pain and reddening of the eyes, swelling of the neck, palpable red swelling and inhibited movement of the fingers; pain, sensation of cold, painful and palpably hot, red swelling in the region of the shoulder and upper arm; lower abdominal pain, migratory abdominal pain, borborygmi, thin stool and excretion of thick, slimy yellow matter; rapid breathing and/or dyspnea; distention swelling & heat along the course of the channel; cold and shivering with an inability to regain warmth; tooth decay, deafness; tooth sensitivity to cold, bi; spasms, stiffness, pain or strain along the course of the channel sinew; inability to raise the arm, inability to turn the neck to the left or right. The LI Channel is most active on Geng days.

Large Intestine Channel

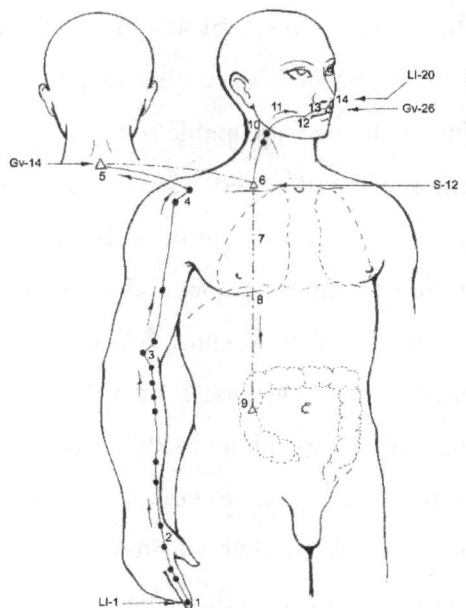

Stomach Channel Symptoms

Borborygmus, abdominal distention, edema, stomachache, vomiting, polyorexia, facial paralysis, sore throat, febrile diseases, mania, pain in the chest, and pain along the course of the channel. This channel also treats excessive brooding or pensiveness. Other signs and symptoms may include high fever or malaria, flushed face, sweating, clouding of the spirit and delirium, manic agitation, aversion to cold, pain in the eyes, dry nose and nosebleed, lesions of the lips and in the mouth, sore larynx, swelling in the neck, dryness of the mouth, chest pain; cold or pain, redness and swelling in the lower limbs; pronounced abdominal distention, fullness and edema; restlessness and discomfort while active or recumbent; or mania and withdrawal; hyperpepsia and quick to hunger; yellow urine; heat in the anterior aspect of the body; persistent hunger, cold in the anterior aspect of the body, shivering, stomach cold resulting in distention and fullness; throat bi, sudden loss of voice; atony of the lower leg muscles; strained middle toe; spasms of the lower leg, hardened muscles in the foot, pain & spasms of the thigh muscles, swellings in the inguinal region, abdominal sinew tension or spasms extending to the neck and jaw, sudden dryness of the mouth; spasms (cold pathogen) with inability to close the eye; heat (pathogen) with inability to open the eye. The Stomach Channel is most active on Wu days.

Stomach Channel

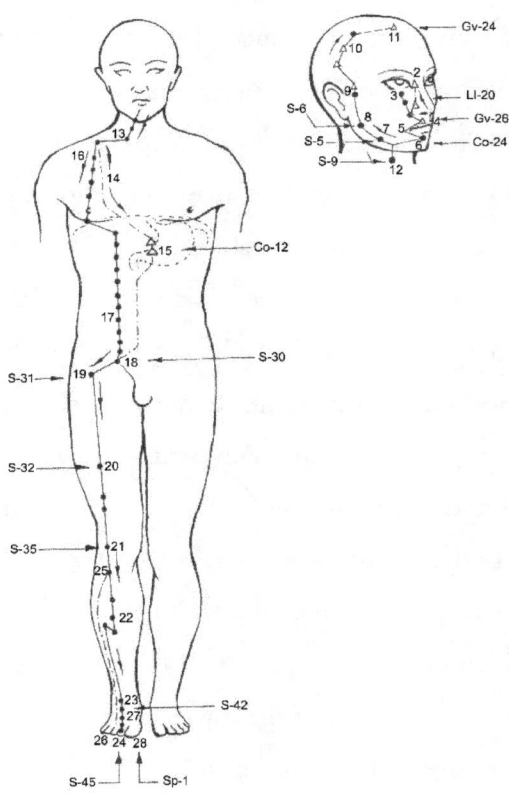

Spleen Channel Symptoms

Abdominal distention, stomachache, diarrhea, dysentery, edema, jaundice, dysuria, lassitude, stiffness and pain in the tongue, pain in the inner side of the thigh and irritability.   Also obsessive thoughts, pensiveness, withdrawal, meditative, contemplative frame of mind. Other signs and symptoms may include heaviness in the head or body, fatigue and weakness of the limbs, general fever, pain in the posterior mandible region and the lower cheek, motor impairment of the tongue, wasting and atony of the muscles of the limbs, cold along the inside of the thigh and knee, edematous swelling of the legs and feet, pain in the abdomen and thin diarrhea or stool containing undigested food, borborygmi, retching and nausea, abdominal lump glomus, reduced food intake, jaundice, inhibited urination, spasm, foot pain, abdominal fullness, intestinal rumbling, untransformed digestate, cholera, cutting pain in the abdomen, drum distension, strain of the large toe, pain at the medial malleolus, cramp and pain in the gastrocnemius, pain in the medial aspect of the knee, pain in the inner thigh and inguinal region, cutting pain in the genitals (this pain may extend up to the navel and ribs or up into the chest or back to the spine), generalized aching and pain, weakness at the limbs and joints. The Spleen Channel is most active during Ji days.

Spleen Channel

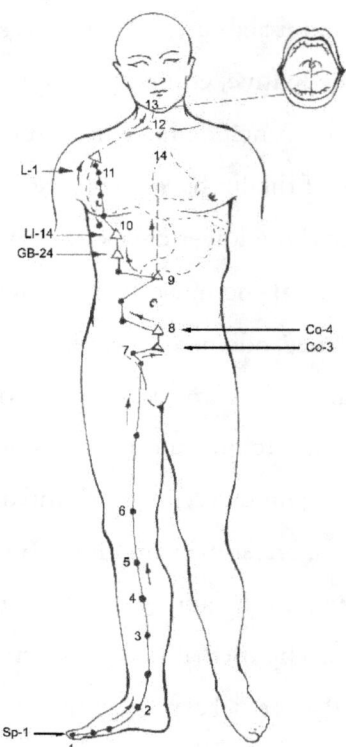

Heart Channel Symptoms

Cardialgia, dry throat, thirst with a desire to drink, yellowish eyeballs, pain in the hypochondriac region and along the channel.   Patients that experience a need to get high, seeking excessive pleasure or joy are also good candidates to be treated with the Heart Channel. Other signs and symptoms may include general fever, headache, pain in the eyes, pain in the chest & back muscles, dry throat, thirst w/ the urge to drink, hot or painful palms, inversion frigidity of the limbs, pain in the scapular region and/or the medial aspect of the forearm, fullness and pain in the chest and lateral costal region, vexation, rapid breathing, discomfort when recumbent, dizziness with fainting spells, Shen disorders, distention and fullness in the region of the diaphragm and chest, inability to speak, internal tension or cramping, pain and cramping as strain along the course of the sinews. The Heart Channel is most active on Ding days.

Heart Channel

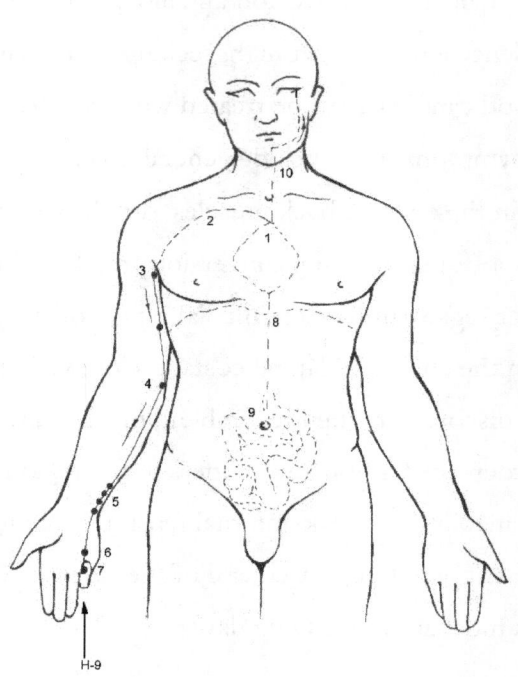

Small Intestine Channel Symptoms

Sore throat, deafness, yellowish eyeballs, swollen cheek, pain in the neck, shoulder, arm and elbow, and other disorders along the running course of the channel. Patients suffering with diseases of the SI Channel may experience restlessness, anxiety, and a sense of foreboding. Other signs and symptoms may include erosion of the glossal and oral mucosa, pain in the cheeks, lachrymation, stiffness of the neck, pain on the lateral aspect of the shoulder and upper arm, lower abdominal pain and distention with the pain stretching around to the lumbar region, lower abdominal pain radiating into the testicles, diarrhea, pain in the stomach with dry feces and constipation, looseness of the joints, atony of the sinews in the elbow region, small wart-like excrescences, strain and inability to support the little finger, pain at the medial aspect of the elbow, the yin aspect of the upper arm and axilla, axillary pain that extends back over the scapula and neck, pain (and tinnitus) in the ear that may extend to the submandibular region, the need to close the eyes for a while to get them to focus, and spasms of tension of the neck sinews resulting in sinew atony or swelling at the neck. The SI Channel is most active on Bing days.

Small Intestine Channel

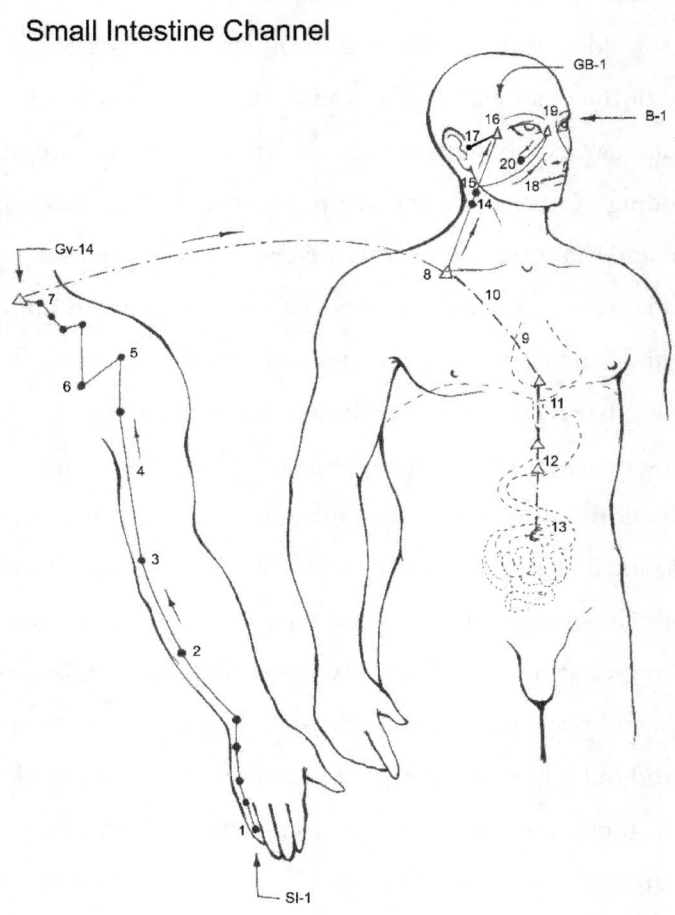

Urinary Bladder Channel Symptoms

Dysuria, enuresis, yellowish eyeballs, epistaxis, headache, mania, pain in the nape, back, lumbar region and along the channel. The patient may have emotional problems of fear, fright, nervousness, anxiousness and anxiety. Other signs and symptoms may include chills & fever, headache, stiff neck, pain in the lumbar region and along the spine, nasal congestion, ocular pain and lacrimation, pain in the posterior thigh, popliteal region, gastrocnemius and foot, pain and distention in the lower abdomen, inhibited micturition, urinary block and enuresis, mental disorders, opisthotonos, nasal congestion with nasal discharge, back pain, nosebleed, strain or inability to support the little toe, pain and swelling of the heel, spasm or tension in the popliteal region, spasm or tension in the neck sinews, inability to raise the arm, muscular discomfort in the axilla, strained muscles in the supraclavicular fossa. The UB Channel is most active on Ren days.

Urinary Bladder Channel

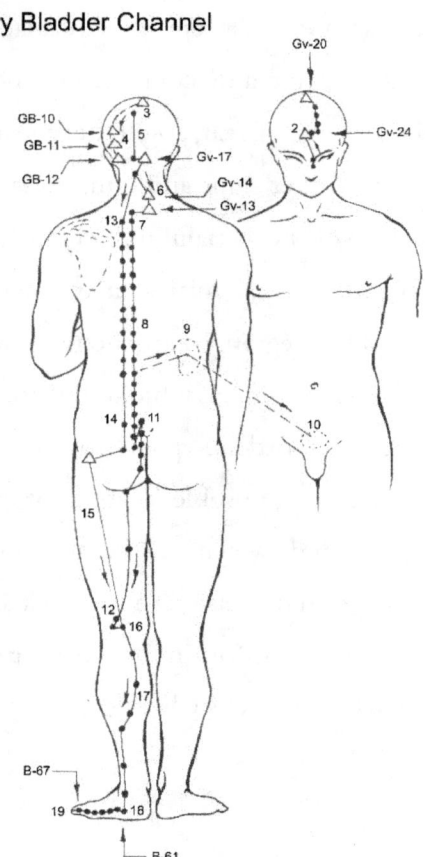

Kidney Channel Symptoms

Hemoptysis, asthma, dry tongue and swollen pharynx, pain in the lumbar region, spinal column and medial side of the thigh, diarrhea, palpitation, and feverish sensation in the center of the sole. The Kidney channel treats fear, fright, nervousness and anxiety. Other signs and symptoms may include counterflow frigidity of the legs, atony of the legs, pain in the lateral gluteal region, pain in the soles of the feet, dizziness, facial edema, bleary eyes, ashen complexion, shortness of breath, short rapid breathing, somnolence or restlessness, enduring diarrhea, thin stool or dry stool evacuated with difficulty, abdominal distention, nausea and vomiting, impotence, blockage of stool and urine, cramping at the bottom of the foot, spasms, twisting or pain along the course of the sinews, convulsions and spasms associated with epileptic diseases. The Kidney Channel is most active during Gui days.

Kidney Channel

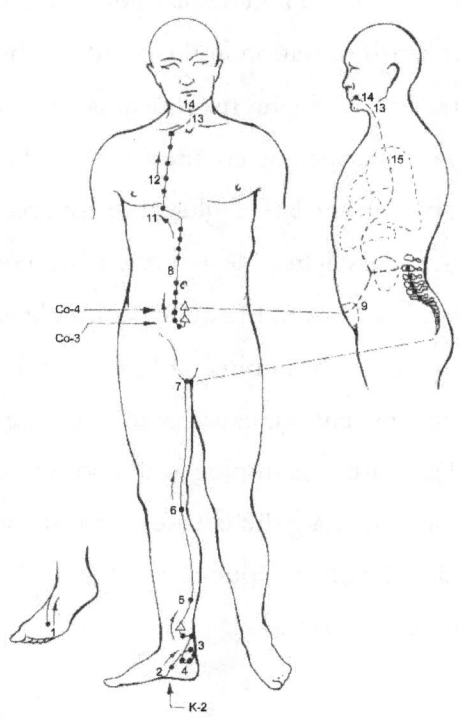

Pericardium Channel Symptoms

Cardialgia, palpitation, irritability, mania, epilepsy, fullness in the chest and hypochondriac region, swollen axilla, spasmodic pain in the elbow and arm, and feverish sensation in the palm. Pericardium protects the heart and houses desires. Other signs and symptoms may include stiffness of the neck, spasm in the limbs, red facial complexion, pain in the eyes, subaxillary swelling, hypertonicity of the elbow and arm inhibiting movement, hot palms, delirious speech, clouding inversion, vexation, fullness and oppression in the chest and lateral costal region, aphasia, palps, cardialgia, constant laughter and other essence-spirit disorders, heart pain, vexation in the heart, spasms, stiffness, strain and pain along the course of the sinews, and chest pain. The Pericardium Channel is most active on Ren days.

Pericardium Channel

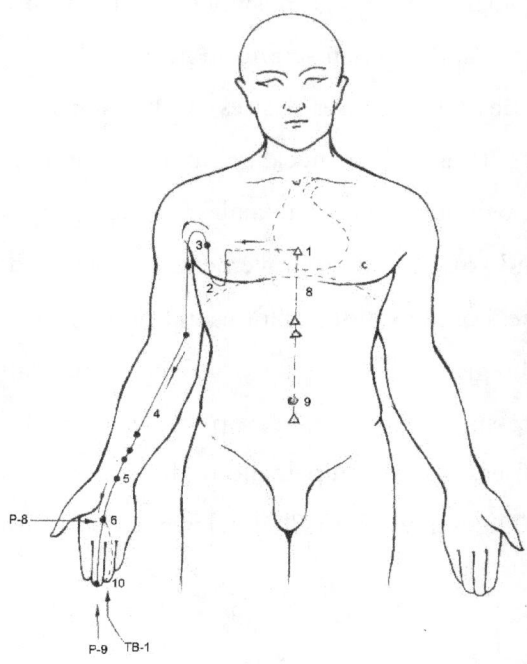

San Jiao Channel Symptoms

Deafness, sweating, sore throat, and other disorders (e.g. pain) in the lateral canthus, cheek, retro-auricular region, shoulder, arm, elbow, and fingers. Other signs and symptoms may include sore throat, pain in the cheeks, reddening of the eyes and eye pain, deafness, pain behind the ears, pain on the posterior aspect of the shoulder and upper arm, abdominal distention and fullness, urinary frequency and distress, vacuity edema of the skin, water swelling, enuresis, spasms and cramps of the muscles around the elbows, atony on the muscles around the elbow, tension and cramps along the course of the sinews and curling of the tongue. The San Jiao Channel is most active on Gui days.

Sanjiao Channel

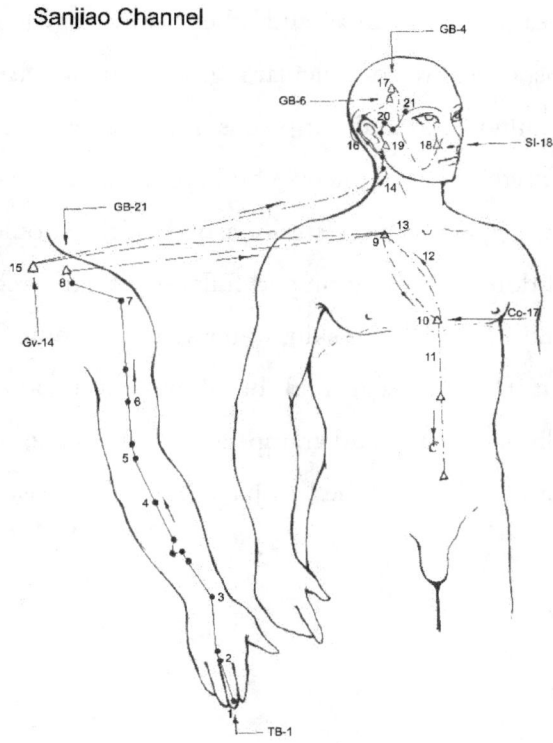

Gall Bladder Channel Symptoms

Bitter taste in mouth, headache, malaria, dizziness, scrofula, swelling in the axillary region, and pain or other disorders in the outer canthus, mandible, supraclavicular fossa, chest, hypochondriac region, thigh and knee. It is said in Chinese Medicine Classics that the Gallbladder is responsible for determination and flexibility. Other signs and symptoms may include alternating fever and chills, headache, malaria, ashen complexion, ocular pain, pain under the chin, subaxillary swelling, scrofulous swellings, deafness, pain in the lateral knee and fibula, pain in the lateral costal area, vomiting, bitter taste in the mouth, pain in the chest, weakness and atony of the lower limbs (with inability to walk and difficulty standing), inability to support the fourth toe, strain and sprains of the outer aspect of the knee, inability to extend and bend the knee, spasm of the popliteal fossa, strains in the pelvic region in the front or the sacro-coccygeal region in the rear, with pain extending up to the lateral costal region or the area just below the lateral costal region, pain in the supraclavicular fossa, the side of the chest or neck, if one looks to the right, the right eye can not remain open and vice versa. The Gallbladder Channel is most active on Jia days.

Gallbladder Channel

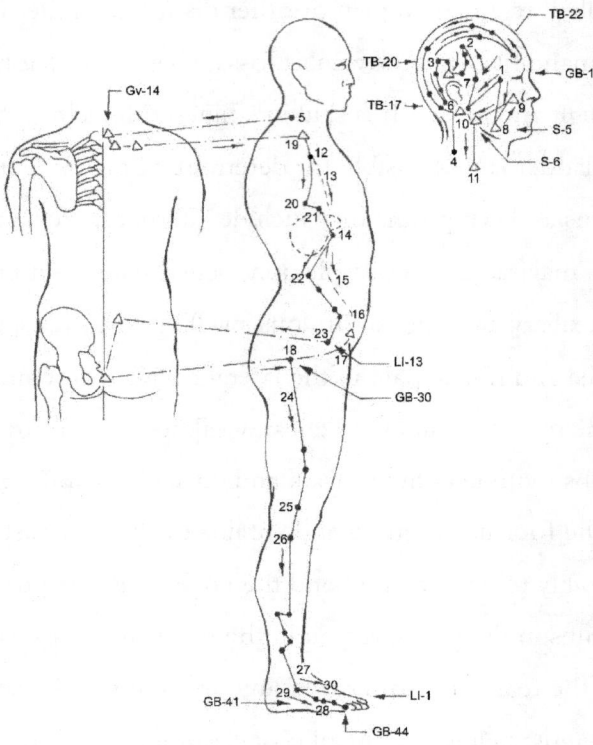

Liver Channel Symptoms

Diarrhea, vomiting, hernia, and enuresis, dysuria, fullness in the chest, swollen lower abdomen, and lumbago.   Since the Liver stores Anger, people suffering from anger should be needled in the Liver Channel. Other signs and symptoms may include dizziness, blurred vision, tinnitus, fever, spasm of the limbs, fullness, distention and pain in the costal region with lump glomus, fullness and thoracic oppression in the abdomen, abdominal pain, vomiting, jaundice, swill (mixture of liquid and solid food) diarrhea, lower abdominal pain, enuresis, urinary block, yellow urine, testicular swelling, frequent erection, fulminant genital itching, inability to support the large toe, pain anterior to the medial malleolus, pain at the medial aspect of the knee, pain or spasm of the medial aspect of the thigh, dysfunction of the genitals, hindered erectile function due to internal damage, retraction of the genitals due to cold damage, and frequent erection due to heat damage. The Liver Channel is most active on Yi days.

Liver Channel

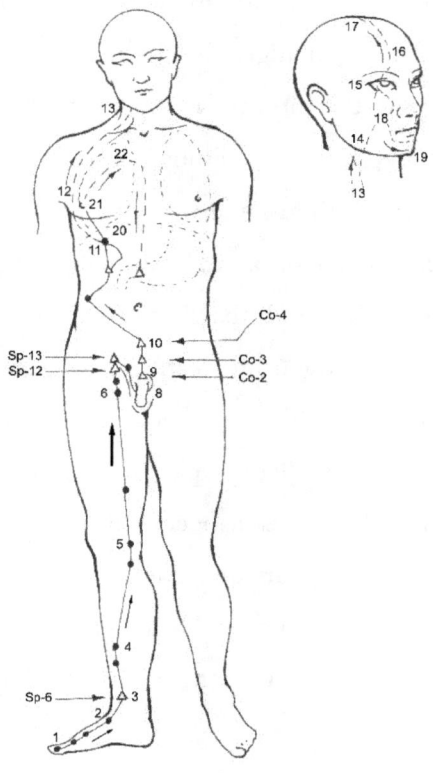

Channel System Methods

Sources: Personal Notes from Lectures by Dr. Young, Robert Chu 2001-2005, **Acupuncturist's Handbook Revised Edition** by Kuen Shii Tsay, Published: 1996, ISBN: 0-9647445-0-3, *Zhong Hua Ji He Xue*, by Liu Yan, Shang Hai Ke Xue Publishing, China 2002, and **Dr. Tan's Strategy of Twelve Magical Points,** Advanced Principles and Techniques in Acupuncture by Richard Tan, self-published 2003, and my own personal notes, Robert Chu, 2001-2004.

In these methods, we are taught to flexibly use channels to relate to each other and choose other channels in lieu of a troubled channel. Knowing these relationships are instrumental in understanding Master Tung's Acupuncture.

Of course, the simplest ways are best. In this text, I use the following Channel methods:

- *Tong Jing Fang Fa – Self Channel Method or Channel related to itself*
- *Tong Ming Jing Fang Fa* - Hand and Foot Channels Method
- *Biao Li Jing Fang Fa* - Interior/Exterior Channel Method
- *Jing Bie Fang Fa* - Branching Channel Method

☯ *Tong Jing Fang Fa* – **Self Channel Method or Channel related to itself**

Every channel can treat itself; for example, if there is a problem with the Stomach channel, *choose* the Stomach channel.

It breaks down as following:

Troubled Channel	Treat with this channel
Lung	Lung
Large Intestine	Large Intestine
Stomach	Stomach
Spleen	Spleen
Heart	Heart
Small Intestine	Small Intestine
Urinary Bladder	Urinary Bladder
Kidney	Kidney
Pericardium	Pericardium
San Jiao	San Jiao
Gall Bladder	Gall Bladder
Liver	Liver

☯ *Tong Ming Jing Fang Fa* - Hand and Foot Channels Method

This is the same channel name relationship, for example, Both the Lung and Spleen are Tai Yin; therefore use the Lung to treat the Spleen. Since the Yang Ming channel is composed of the Large Intestine and Stomach Channels, use them to treat each other.

This breaks down as:

Troubled Channel	Treat with this channel
Lung	Spleen
Large Intestine	Stomach
Stomach	Large Intestine
Spleen	Lung
Heart	Kidney
Small Intestine	Urinary Bladder
Urinary Bladder	Small Intestine
Kidney	Heart
Pericardium	Liver
San Jiao	Gall Bladder
Gall Bladder	San Jiao
Liver	Pericardium

☯ *Biao Li Jing Fang Fa* - **Interior/Exterior Channel Method**

This is the common Internal -external relationship as found in TCM. For example, use Lung Channel to treat the Large Intestine Channel. The rest follow accordingly.

This breaks down as:

Troubled Channel	Treat with this channel
Lung	Large Intestine
Large Intestine	Lung
Stomach	Spleen
Spleen	Stomach
Heart	Small Intestine
Small Intestine	Heart
Urinary Bladder	Kidney
Kidney	Urinary Bladder
Pericardium	San Jiao
San Jiao	Pericardium
Gall Bladder	Liver
Liver	Gall Bladder

☯ *Jing Bie Fang Fa* - Branching Channel Method

This method is alternatively known as the *Zang Fu Bei Tong* theory and was expounded by Dr, Young Wei-chieh. Dr. Tan presented this information as *"Bie Jing"* System.

This theory stems from the *Nei Jing* and *Ling Shu* and shows how diseases progress from exterior to interior. It was later modified by Zhang Zhong Jing in his text *Shang Han Lun* (Discussion of Cold Induced Diseases) on herbal formulae. The root of this theory is expounded in the *Yi Jing* (Classic of Changes), where one trigram is put on top of another forming a hexagram. A trigram is said to have three layers – if we take a yang trigram (*Qian Gua*), the outermost layer is *Tai Yang*, the middle layer is *Shao Yang*, and the root or base layer is *Yang Ming*. If we take a Yin Trigram (*Kun Gua*), there are also three layers, the upper most is *Tai Yin*, the middle is *Shao Yin*, the bottom layer, *Jue Yin*. From here, if they are transposed on top of each other, they show a relationship of Upper, Middle and Lower. In the Nei Jing, this is referred to as the *Guan, Shu, He* relationship. There are 3 sets of Branching relationship for the channels: *Tai Yang* and *Tai Yin* treat each other, *Shao Yang and Shao Yin* treat each other, *Yang Ming* and *Jue Yin* treat each other.

This breaks down as:

Troubled Channel	Treat with this channel
Lung	Small Intestine or Urinary Bladder
Large Intestine	Pericardium or Liver
Stomach	Pericardium or Liver
Spleen	Small Intestine or Urinary Bladder
Heart	San Jiao or Gall Bladder
Small Intestine	Lung or Spleen
Urinary Bladder	Lung or Spleen
Kidney	San Jiao or Gall Bladder
Pericardium	Large Intestine or Stomach
San Jiao	Heart or Kidney
Gall Bladder	Heart or Kidney
Liver	Large Intestine or Stomach

Methods involving Time and Channels

Here we introduce Methods involving Time and Channels. We make use of the Chinese Shi Chen (2 Hour) methods, and the use of the Stems and branches.

Prior to the Qing Dynasty, the Chinese used a different method to keep track of time, day, month, seasons and year. They used the Stems and Branches. There are Ten Stems that *include jia, yi, bing, ding, wu, ji, geng, xin, ren,* and *gui.* In the Diseased channels section of the book, I explain which days the channel system is most active. We also make use of the twelve branches, *zi, chou, yin, mao, chen, si, wu, wei, shen, you, xu,* and *hai.*

As this is a Primer, the subject matter is too expansive, so I just include a brief introduction here. Here, I show 3 methods of using ChronoAcupuncture:

☯ **Horary Point with Mother or Son Method**
☯ *Zi Wu Fang Fa* **- Hour Channel Method**
☯ *Liu Zhu Fang Fa* **- Ebb and Flow Channel Method**

☯ **Horary Point with Mother or Son**

In this method, we use the open channel of the time (Shi Chen) and choose the appropriate Ben (Horary) point, and Mu (Mother) or Zi (Son) point. Of course, as acupuncturists, we learn to use the Mother point for tonification, and the Son for sedation. The use of the Horary point is to affect the channel in general.

Time	*Shi Chen*	Channel	*Ben*	*Mu/Zi*
11 pm – 1 am	*Zi*	GB	GB41	GB 43/38
1 - 3 am	*Chou*	Liv	Liv 1	Liv 8/2
3 - 5 am	*Yin*	Lu	Lu 8	Lu 9/5
5 - 7 am	*Mao*	LI	LI 1	LI 11/2
7 - 9 am	*Chen*	St	St 36	St 41/45
9 – 11 am	*Si*	Sp	Sp 3	Sp 2/5
11am – 1pm	*Wu*	H	H 8	H 9/7
1 – 3 pm	*Wei*	SI	SI 5	SI 3/8
3 –5 pm	*Shen*	UB	UB 66	UB 67/65
5 – 7 pm	*You*	K	K 10	K 7/1
7 – 9 pm	*Xu*	Pc	Pc 8	Pc 9/7
9 – 11 pm	*Hai*	SJ	SJ 6	SJ 3/10

☯ *Zi Wu Fang Fa* - Hour Channel Method

In ancient China, months and hours were named after the earthly branches. We still use the Chinese hours in *Feng Shui*, *Ba Zi* (horoscope) and acupuncture. We can use the hours, called *Shi Chen* to correspond to the current clock. One *Shi Chen* is equal to two standard hours. These relate to the organs and channels.

Shi Chen	Organ	Hours
Zi	Gall Bladder	23 hour to 01 hour
Chou	Liver	01 hour to 03 hour
Yin	Lung	03 hour to 05 hour
Mao	Large Intestine	05 hour to 07 hour
Chen	Stomach	07 hour to 09 hour
Si	Spleen	09 hour to 11 hour
Wu	Heart	11 hour to 13 hour
Wei	Small Intestine	13 hour to 15 hour
Shen	Urinary Bladder	15 hour to 17 hour
You	Kidney	17 hour to 19 hour
Xu	Pericardium	19 hour to 21 hour
Hai	San Jiao	21 hour to 23 hour

Because the 12 Earthly Stems have an a.m. – p.m. relationship, we can also arrange them as:

Zi	*Chou*	*Yin*	*Mao*	*Chen*	*Si*
Wu	*Wei*	*Shen*	*You*	*Xu*	*Hai*

This is why we refer to them as the *Zi Wu* System. Dr. Tan taught this simplified as the "Opposite Clock System", but this has a long history in China, in an acupuncture system called *Zi Wu Liu Zhu* (Ebb and Flow of 12 Branches Time), a part of classical acupuncture. We can also use this method to choose channels. When there is a troubled channel, we can choose the opposite time to treat the troubled channel.

GB	Liv	Lu	LI	St	Sp
H	SI	UB	K	Pc	SJ

This can break down more simply as:

Troubled Channel	**Treat with this channel**
Lung	Urinary Bladder
Large Intestine	Kidney
Stomach	Pericardium
Spleen	San Jiao
Heart	Gall Bladder
Small Intestine	Liver
Urinary Bladder	Lung
Kidney	Large Intestine
Pericardium	Stomach
San Jiao	Spleen
Gall Bladder	Heart
Liver	Small Intestine

For those of you who like a simpler image that looks more similar to the Chinese clock, we have shaded the hours for P.M. and left A.M. as unshaded:

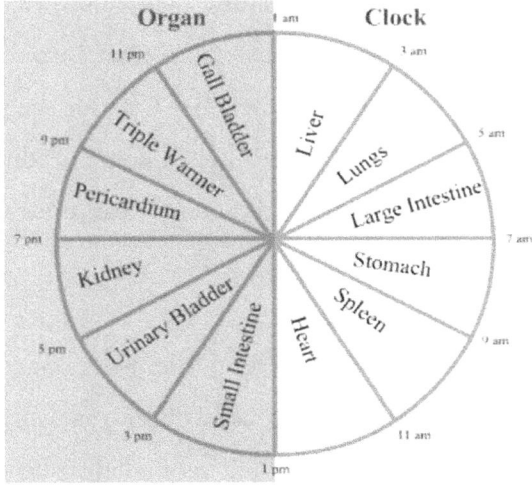

☯ *Liu Zhu Fang Fa* - **Ebb and Flow Channel Method**

In ancient China, the old acupuncture system called *Zi Wu Liu Zhu* (Ebb and Flow of 12 Branches Time), allowed us to be flexible to choose channels. Since all the channels ebb and flow into each other, we can make use of these relationships to treat a troubled channel. Many simply choose to treat the next *Shi Chen*, or the next channel. This, however, is a very simplified way. Energy is constantly ebbing and flowing for all the channels, as such we can draw upon the relations between the channels.

If we borrow a concept from the Five Elements concepts, we know that every channel has a "Mother" and "Son", as well as "Grandmother" and "Grandson". These relationships may be exploited to treat a troubled channel. It is like a family, coming to aid for a relative. For example, The Liver might be considered the "Mother" of the Lungs, the Large Intestine as the "Son" of the Lungs. The Gall Bladder might be considered as "Grand Mother" of the Lungs, and the Stomach as the "Grandson". In this way, we can exploit those relationships fully and we may or may not include the troubled channel in our treatments.

The late Richard Tan taught this method as the "Neighbor Clock System", but only used a simplified version.

From reflection, we can see that acupuncture, especially in the Chrono Acupuncture sense, is a very mysterious subject, and I will be writing more about this in my forthcoming book on ChronoAcupuncture.

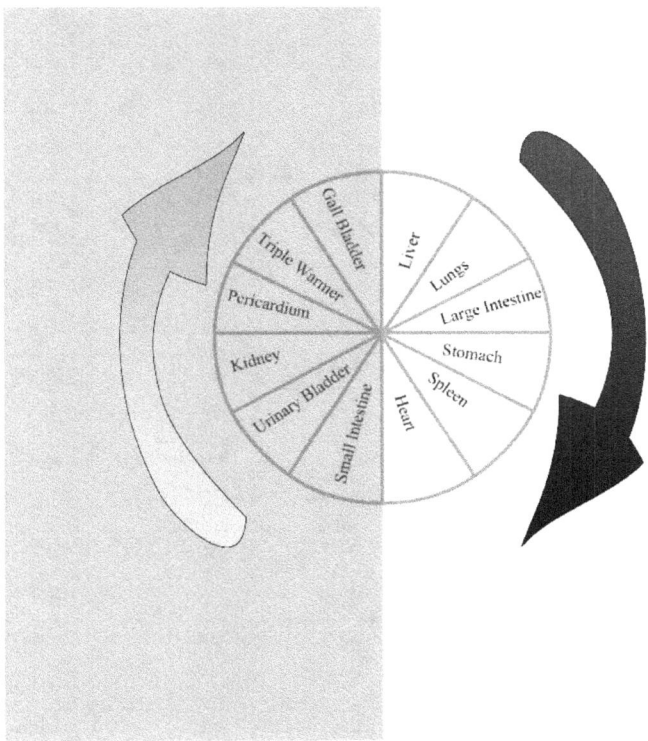

We can break this down as follows:

Troubled Channel	Son Channel	Mother Channel	Grandson Channel	Grand Mother
Lung	Large Intestine	Liver	Stomach	Gall Bladder
Large Intestine	Stomach	Lung	Spleen	Liver
Stomach	Spleen	Large Intestine	Heart	Lung
Spleen	Heart	Stomach	Small Intestine	Large Intestine
Heart	Small Intestine	Spleen	Urinary Bladder	Stomach
Small Intestine	Urinary Bladder	Heart	Kidney	Spleen
Urinary Bladder	Kidney	Small Intestine	Pericardium	Heart
Kidney	Pericardium	Urinary Bladder	San Jiao	Small Intestine
Pericardium	San Jiao	Kidney	Gall Bladder	Urinary Bladder
San Jiao	Gall Bladder	Pericardium	Liver	Kidney
Gall Bladder	Liver	San Jiao	Lung	Pericardium
Liver	Lung	Gall Bladder	Large Intestine	San Jiao

This chart alone differentiates many ways of selecting channels to aid the troubled channel. This can also help use when we combine channels in circuits, but I have already explained that in my book, **The Best of Master Tung's Acupuncture**.

☯ IMAGING METHODS

Sources: *Zhen Jiu Jing Wei*, by Young Wei-Chieh, Zhi Yuan Publishing, Taiwan 1985, ISBN: 957-8609-43-4 and *Taiwan Dong Shi Zhen Jiu Shou Jiao Dui Ying Zhen Fa*, by Li Guo Zhen, Zhi Yuan Publishing, Taiwan 1996

Introduction

This is a unique feature of Master Tung's acupuncture. This method as it is extrapolated in the *Su Wen* Chapter 63 where it discusses needling from the opposite side. When combined with the theory of the *Ba Gua* (Eight Diagrams), we can extrapolate eight basic methods. The imaging method shows a method of corresponding one part of the body with another part of the body. We may apply this principle to create new uses of the 14 channel points. This core concept explains why there are so many points and how to use all acupoints flexibly.

These don't have to be remembered by rote memorization. You can have fun with them. Stick to one Imaging Method first, then master them, one by one. Start with the first eight basic methods, then move onto the Advanced methods. When you have imaging and you have channels, you have a point. You don't have to be limited to Classical points or Master Tung's points, you can make up your own points if you want, just avoid dangerous or anatomical areas.

In treatment of all diseases, you first select and identify the troubled channel, then apply the imaging method, then insert the needles. The channel is the longitude, the imaging is the latitude. When you have longitude and latitude, you have a point. This is then time to introduce the needle(s). This can be used flexibly with the myriad ways of channels which are interrelated, and the myriad ways of Imaging.

In this way, acupuncture becomes fun, creative, more exciting to see what the outcomes are. Of course, your practice will grow as you observe greater clinical results.

Of these imaging methods, the most commonly used ones in the clinic are Same Height imaging, Hand and Foot Imaging, Hand and Torso Imaging, Foot and Torso Imaging, and Flipped Imaging.

☯ Same Height Imaging

In this method, points that correspond on the same plane can be chosen to treat a particular disease. For example, pain at the elbow at LI11 may be treated with the opposite side Lu 5. Another example would be that Ren 24 may be used to treat occipital neck pain.

I have summarized this in this chart:

Affected Area	Then Treat Opposite Side:
Left side of head	Head
Left Ear	Ear
Left Neck	Neck
Left Shoulder	Shoulder
Left Breast	Breast
Left Abdomen	Abdomen
Left Low Back	Low Back
Left Hip	Hip
Left Knee	Knee
Left Ankle	Ankle
Left Top of Foot	Top of Foot
Left Heel	Heel

☯ Hand and Foot Imaging

In this method, the foot is treated by the hand and vice versa; the ankle is treated by the wrist; the lower leg corresponds to the forearm; the knee corresponds to the elbow; and the thigh corresponds to the upper arm.

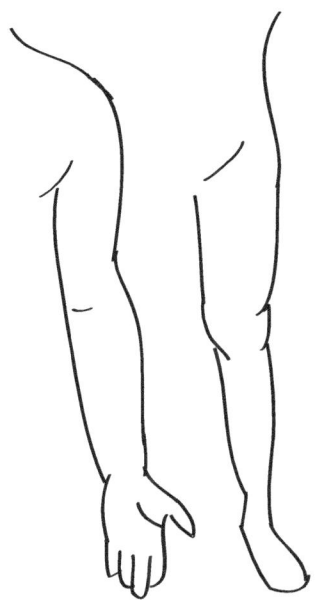

We can break this down as follows:

Arm	Leg
Shoulder	Hip
Upper Arm	Thigh
Elbow	Knee
Forearm	Lower Leg
Wrist	Ankles
Hand	Foot
Fingers	Toes
Palms	Sole

☯ Hand and Foot Opposite Imaging

In this method, the foot corresponds to the shoulder; the lower leg corresponds to the upper arm; the elbows and knees correspond; the thigh corresponds to the forearm.

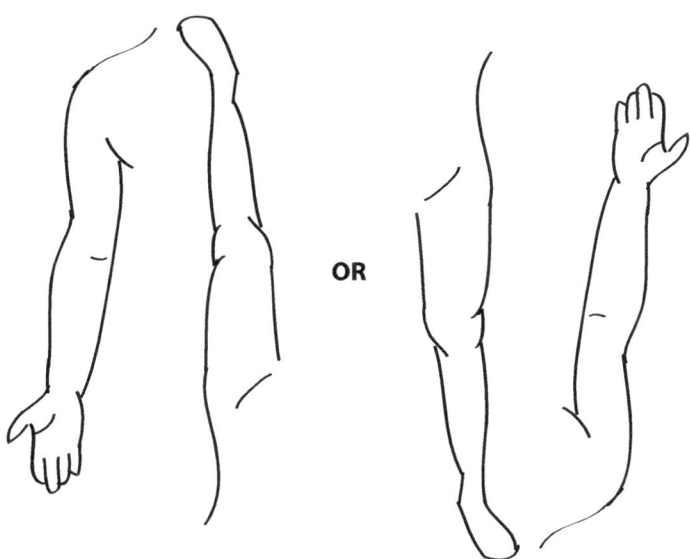

We can break this down as follows:

Arm	Leg
Shoulder	Soles
Upper Arm	Lower Legs
Elbow	Knee
Forearm	Thighs
Wrist	Hips
Hand	Pelvic Area
Fingers	Groin Area
Palms	Hips

☯ Hand and Torso Imaging

In this method, the neck corresponds to the wrist, chest to the forearm, and umbilicus to the elbow, groin to the shoulder, An example illustrating this would be for neck pain, use SJ 5, Lu5, LI5

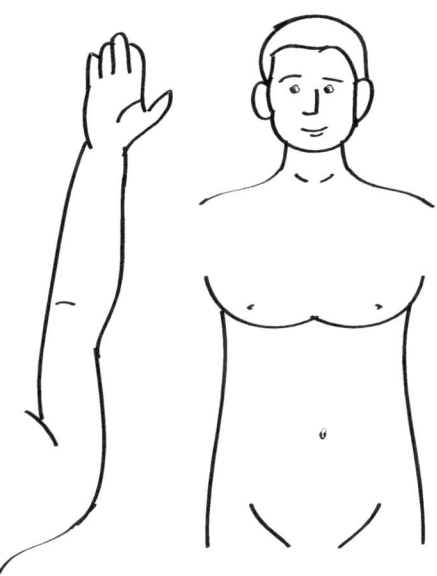

We can break this down as follows:

Arm	Body
Fingers	Scalp/Top of Head
Palm	Face
Back of Hand	Occipital region
Wrist	Neck
Forearm	Chest
Elbow	Abdominal Area
Upper Arm	Lower Abdomen
Shoulders	Groin

☯ Hand and Torso Opposite Imaging

In this method, the arm and torso are flipped.

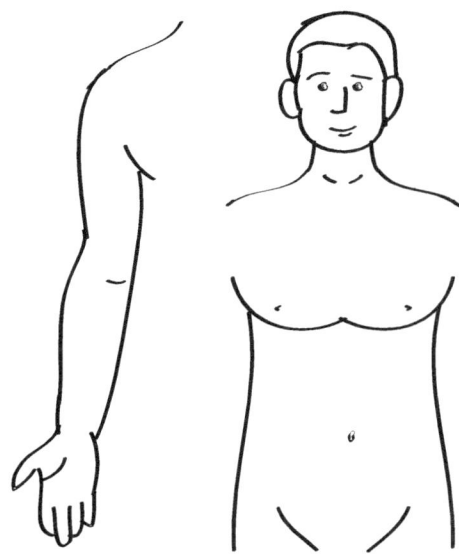

We can break this down as follows:

Arm	Head and Torso
Shoulder	Head and Neck
Upper Arm	Shoulders and Chest
Elbow	Umbilicus
Forearm	Abdomen
Wrist	Hips
Hand	Pelvic Area
Fingers	Groin Area

☯ Foot and Torso Imaging

With this method, we would use the Foot to treat facial problems, ankle to treat neck problems, lower leg to treat chest problems. The rest may be inferred.

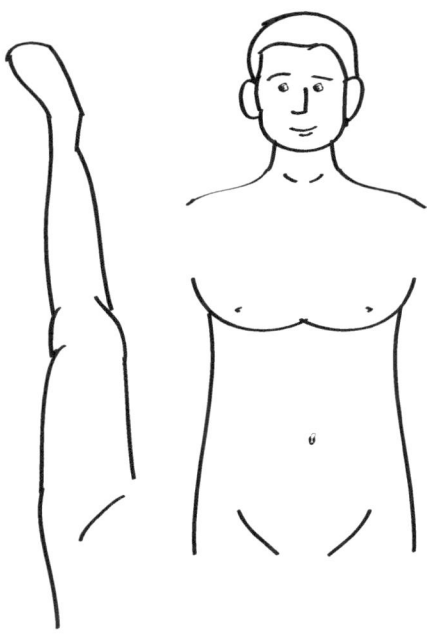

We can break this down as follows:

Foot	Torso
Toes	Head
Foot	Face
Ankle	Neck
Lower Leg	Chest
Knee	Umbilicus
Thigh	Abdomen
Top of Thigh	Pelvic Region
Hip	Groin

☯ Foot and Torso Opposite Imaging

In this method, for neck problems, we needle the thigh, for the lower abdomen, we use the lower leg. An example of this would be for impotence use Liv 1, or for Stomach problems, use St 36

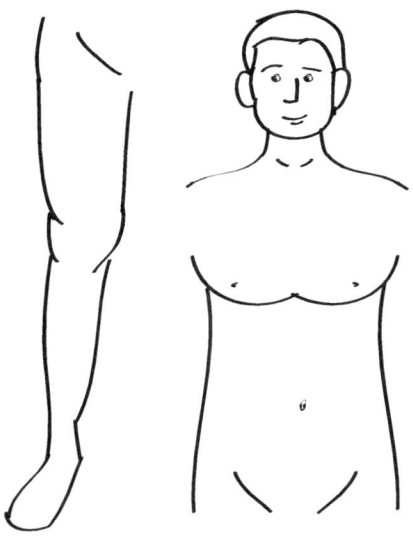

We can break this down as follows:

Leg	Torso
Hip	Head
Pelvic Area	Neck
Thigh	Chest
Knee	Umbilicus
Lower Leg	Abdominal Region
Ankles	Lower Abdomen
Foot	Groin Area
Toes	Groin
Sole	Perineum

☯ Flipped Imaging

In this method, we think of a torso overlayed and a flipped image of it on the torso. Examples to illustrate this method would be LI 20 for worms, or pain in the perineum we needle Du 26

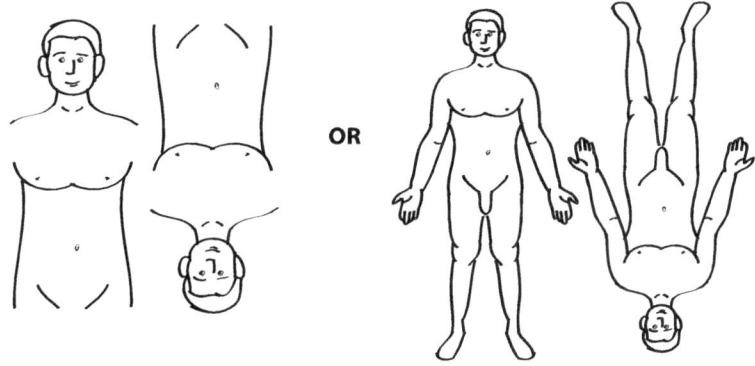

We can break this down as follows:

Torso to Flipped Torso Illustration:

Head	Buttocks
Face	Groin
Neck	Lower Abdomen
Chest	Abdomen
Abdomen	Chest
Lower Abdomen	Face
Pubic Region	Forehead
Groin	Nose
Perineum	Top of head

Body/Inverted BodyIllustration:

Part of Body	Corresponds to
Head	Feet
Neck	Ankles
Chest	Ankles/Lower Legs
Abdomen	Knees
Lower Abdomen	Groin
Thighs	Lower Abdomen
Knees	Chest
Lower Legs	Chest
Ankles	Neck
Feet	Face
Toes	Top of Head

Of course, there are many other methods of imaging , and whole systems which we call holographs (*Quan Xi*, in Chinese), but that is beyond the scope of this Primer.

☯ Exercises to enhance understanding –

What would we choose for neck pain?

How could we treat a sprained ankle?

What part of the face would we needle if a patient is suffering from pain in the penis?

ADVANCED IMAGING METHODS

Source: © Robert Chu, November 2005

Introduction

When one looks more and more into the Master Tung Acupuncture system, we see more and more that there are multiple layers of imaging. Here, we will examine more of the advanced imaging methods.

Of these Advanced imaging methods, the most commonly used ones in the clinic are Forearm images the Torso, Whole Body, Thigh, Lower Leg and upper arm imaging, and Lower Leg images the Torso, Whole Body, Thigh, upper arm, and forearm imaging . This gives us an insight into why our ancestors usually needled below the knees and below the elbows.   In addition, the most powerful points, the antique points which have over 2500 years of written history, reside below the elbows and knees.

In my own clinic, I use the Imaging methods of the Lower Leg images the Torso, Whole Body, Thigh, upper arm, and Forearm images the Torso, Whole Body, Thigh, upper arm and Lower Leg imaging most.

Many of my students who own "community style" acupuncture clinics also find it most convenient to use these points.

☯ Forearm images the Torso, Whole Body, Thigh, Lower Leg and upper arm imaging

In this method, the forearm is the reference point to image the other portions of the body, and referred points on the same plane can be chosen to treat a particular disease. For example, headache can be treated by needling points around the elbow. Another example would be hip pain can be treated by needling the fingers.

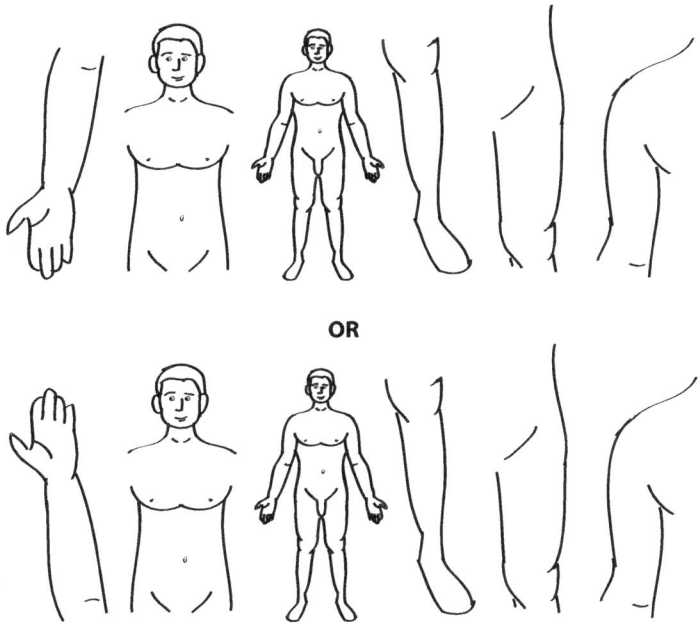

☯ Lower Leg images the Torso, Whole Body, Thigh, upper arm, and forearm imaging

In this method, the lower leg is the reference point to treat referred portions of the body. An example would be needling the knee at St 35 to treat sinus problems, or using GB 34 to treat hip pain.

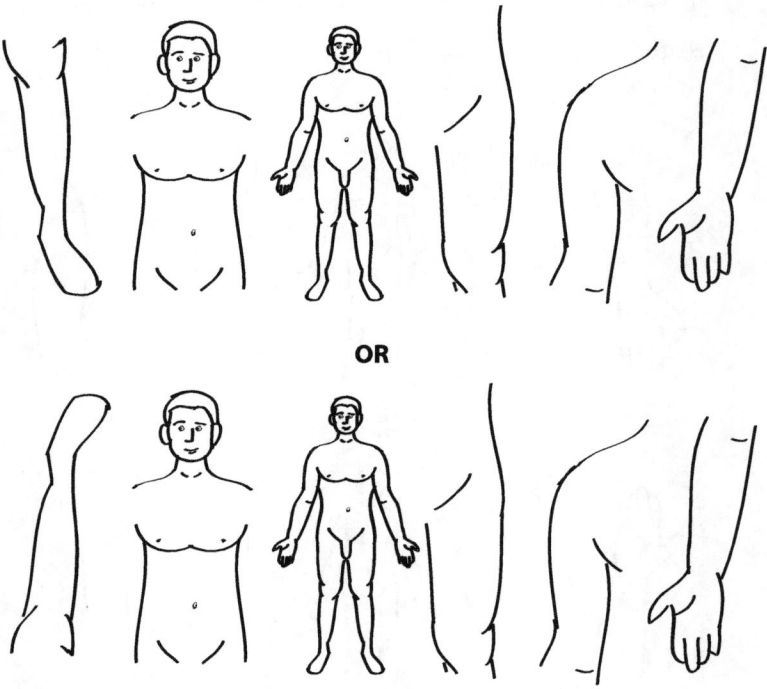

OR

☯ Upper Leg images the Torso, Whole Body, Lower Leg, upper arm, and forearm imaging

In this method, the Upper leg/Thigh can be used to treat referred areas. An example of this is using the thigh points to treat stomach problems, or abdominal problems, as in Master Tung's *Si Ma San* and *Ming Huang* points. Another example would be using GB 31 to treat forearm pain.

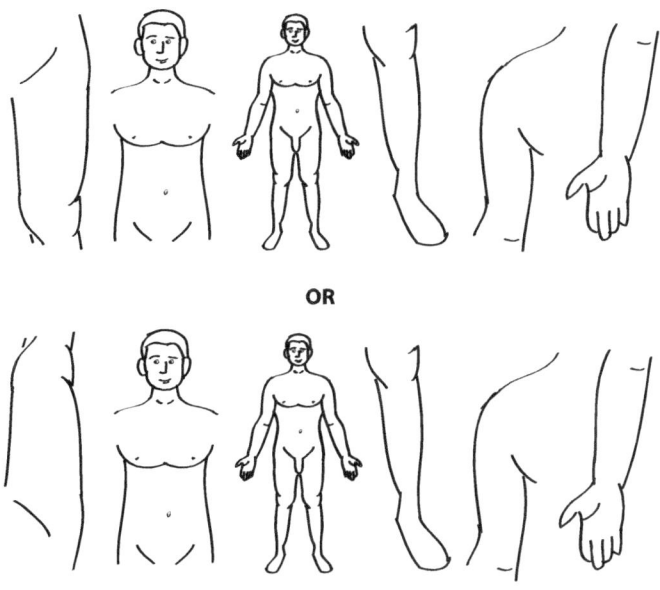

OR

☯ Upper Arm images Torso, Whole Body, Upper leg, Lower leg and forearm imaging

In this method, the upper arm is the reference point to use as an image to treat corresponding areas. An example illustrating this would be needling the shoulder to treat knee pain as in Master Tung's *Jian Zhong* point.

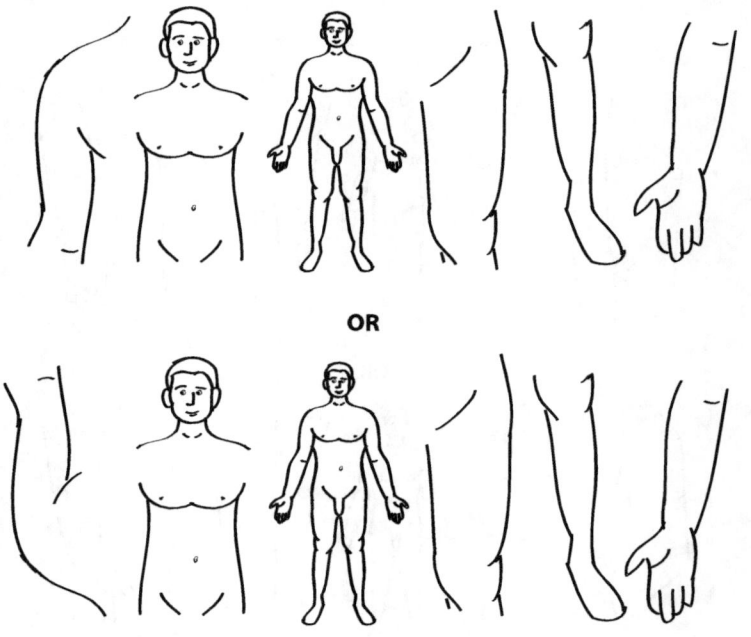

OR

☯ Exercises to enhance understanding –

How would you treat ankle pain now?

What would you needle to treat neck pain?

Can the images be flipped from ventral to dorsal and flipped vertically for other referred areas?

Other Methods of Point Location

In knowing the channels and knowing the imaging you can create points to treat diseases.

Palpation skills and knowledge of the physical location of the points is necessary. Palpation skills are a part of the physical medicine of acupuncture. We have to be great at topical anatomy and learn through year of mentoring and practice in the clinic. It is a great shame that many of today's acupuncturists no longer have to take a practical examination, in person, to demonstrate proficiency in palpation, location, and needling skills.

I want to pass this oral tradition to the readers of this book – use your fingertips first to get a general location and feel of a point from a topical anatomy point of view, but before inserting needles, use your fingernail to palpate the area.

The next few chapters explain a combination of channels and imaging.

- ☯ *Ashi Xue Wei Fang Fa* – "That's It!" Point Method
- ☯ *San Guan Fang Fa* – Three Passes Point Location Method
- ☯ *Wu Shu Xue Fang Fa* – Antique Points Point Location methods
- ☯ *Zhang Ying Qing* Holographic Method

☯ *Ashi Xue Wei Fang Fa* – That's It! Point Method

The *Ashi Xue Wei Fang Fa* is one of the easiest methods of acupuncture. *Ashi* is a method coined Sun Si Miao (581-682 A.D.), a famous physician, who wrote the *Qian Jin Yao* Fang (Thousand Ducat Formulas), "In the method of *ashi*, with a person who has pain, we can palpate (the channels), and the patient will reply, "*A Shi!*" (literally, "Ah, yes!" or "That's it!") . His logic was simple - We cannot ask a layman if so-and –so point is a known acupuncture point.

For those who are unfamiliar with points, and are more kinesthetic in their approach and prefer to palpate for points, this is your way. The other methods presuppose that you know acupuncture points and channels and how they are located. In this method, you simply palpate along the channels to find your points. But you must know your channel pathways in general.

Channels are often described as a thickness of 2 mm in width. I prefer not to use his method in width of the channel. In my paradigm of acupuncture, I simple state the channel is one sixth of your limb. In stating as such, channels are pretty thick. Many would consider what I do as the tendino-muscular meridians. That is fine. My area of activation is very wide. My points are also bigger than most people would be accustomed to. As I mentioned earlier, by using the channels and imaging, you have both "longitude" and "latitude", and therefore, you would have a "point". This is the simplest way to find points, and actually the most accurate. Japanese acupuncture specializes in this method, and the famous Chinese Acupuncturist, Wang Ju Yi, is famous for his palpation methods.

I highly recommend this way when you are both starting out or already an accomplished acupuncturist. For the beginner, it can help you find the points. For the advanced practitioner, it can help you cut down on points. For example, through palpation of *Ashi* points, you could actually just needle two out of three points which are the more sensitive.

☯ *San Guan Fang Fa* – Three Passes Point Location Method

In this method, I use a term borrowed from one of the famous Master Tung's set of points called Wai San Guan 外 三 關 – External Three Gates or Passes. This is a *Dao Ma* (footnote 1) or *Hui Ma* set of points. Master Tung taught *Dao Ma Zhen* 倒 馬 針(Fallen Horse Needling) or what is known as *Hui Ma Zhen* 回馬針(Returning Horse Needling) as a technique unique to Master Tung's Acupuncture in where needling is performed in succession to emphasize a particular channel and send a signal to the brain to restore the body in harmony.

Needling here is done in three's, like the childrens' game of "tic-tac-toe, 3 in a row". The idea is to send a signal strong enough in the body to not be ignored. Sometimes, in *Dao Ma* method, we use just a paired set of points.

If we just use a coupled set of points these would represent upper and lower, or Heaven and Earth. Whereas in the Three needle technique represents Heaven, Human, and Earth – the *San Cai* 三才or 3 Primordial relations.

1) This has been a subject of study by Dr. Young Wei-chieh in his seminal work, **Dong Si Qi Xue Zhen Jiu Xue**, *Zhi Yuan* Publishing, Taiwan in 1992, and Lee Kuo-chen's (aka Li Guo Zhen) **Taiwan Dong Si Zhen Jiu Dao Ma Zhen Ci Liao Fa**, Zhi Yuan Publishing, Taiwan in 1994, and **Advanced Tung Style Acupuncture: The Dao Ma Needling Technique of Master**

Tung Ching-Chang by James H. Maher, DC, OMD, Dipl,Ac., self-published, in 2004, ISBN 0-9759096-9-X.

Wai San Guan is located as 3 points on the Gallbladder Channel, start by drawing an imaginary line between the head of the fibula and the tip of the lateral malleolus, the 2nd point is the mid-point, the upper point is the midpoint between the 2nd point and the head of the fibula; the lower point is the midpoint between the 2nd point and the tip of the lateral malleolus.

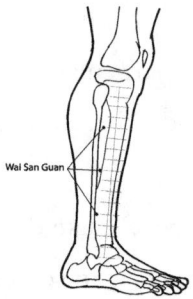

Master Tung used *Wai San Guan* traditionally for shoulder pain, upper arm pain, tonsillitis, frozen shoulder, acne, tumors, Pneumonia, Lateral Forearm Pain, Mumps, Adenofibroma of the Breast, Laryngitis, Benign neoplasm of thyroid gland, Goiter, hypothyroidism, Obesity, Forearm Pain, Reflexive Sympathy Disorder, Parkinson's Disease, and low back pain.

My introducing *Wai San Guan* here is to use the idea of *Wai San Guan,* but not necessarily the *Hui Ma* point combination. You start by drawing an imaginary line between the upper epicondyle of a bone and the lower epicondyle of a bone, the 2nd point is the mid- point, the upper point is the midpoint between the 2nd point and the head of the bone; the lower point is the midpoint between the 2nd point and the tip of the tail of the bone. You simply apply this model of three points on every long bone of the body.

You can apply the "Three Passes" on any channel on the lower or upper limbs. This way, you automatically have a Dao Ma set on each channel, and I simply call them in English as "Such and Such Channel Three Passes" or "In-between Channels Three Passes", leading an acupuncturist to create their own Dao Ma sets.

☯ *Wu Shu Xue Fang Fa* – Antique Point Location Method

The Antique points have the longest recorded written history of use in the classics, and area micro system unto themselves. In this method, we use the Antique points to locate the important points that we need along a channel to treat. We simply apply the logic of imaging and use the Antique points to treat. The Antique points are located between he fingers or toes and below the elbows or knees respectively. They are already linked towards different parts of the body based on their indications. There are many classical indications of the Antique points:

In Classical Acupuncture, we consider the use of them as the most powerful points on the arms and legs, below the elbows and below the knees.

The *Jing* Well points are used for mental problems or delirium. The *Nan Jing* states the *Jing* Well Points are for "fullness below the heart". The *Jia Yi Jing* states that these *Jing* Well points are for problems in the viscera. To treat any Liver related channel problems, we choose the *Jing* Well Points.

Ying Spring points are used for "fever in the upper part of the body" according to the *Nan Jing*, or for "Body heat". The *Jia Yi Jing* states that the *Ying* Spring points are for changes in color. I like to state these are used for any type of *"-itis"* (inflammation). The *Ying* Spring points are used for Heart Problems, in the summer time, and also treat vessel problems.

The *Shu* Stream points are for "pain and heaviness in the body, and joint pain" according to the *Nan Jing*. The *Jia Yi Jing* states that these *Shu* Stream points are for problems that alternate mild and severe. They are most active in the Late Summer, which means they can be used all year long. They are used to treat Spleen Channel problems.

Yuan Source points move the qi along the channels and meridians. They are in control of the *Qi* of the *San jiao* and control the *Yuan Qi* in the channels. If one needs to activate the channels, the *Yuan* Source point is utilized.

Luo Connecting points transfer qi from one channel to another channel. In TCM acupuncture, they are used to transfer qi from the internal and externally related channels, for example, the Lung to the Large Intestine. In Optimal Acupuncture, because we are very flexible in the interrelationships of the channels, we know we can always direct qi to an affected channel through the use of the *Luo* connecting points.

Xi Cleft points are underutilized in TCM Acupuncture. The *Xi* Cleft points are used for any type of pain and bleeding. They are our trauma points, used for any pain, whether acute or chronic.

Jing River points are used for "cough, and alternating hot and cold disease" according to the *Nan Jing*. The *Jia Yi Jing* states that the *Jing* River points are for changes in the voice, and fullness in the channels or *Luo*. *Jing* River points are used in the Autumn season and treat the Lung channel problems.

He Sea points are used for "reversal of Qi and Diarrhea" and are pricked in the Winter according to the *Nan Jing*. The *Jia Yi Jing* states that the *He* Sea points are for problems in the stomach and chest. They are used for treating the Kidney channel, and to connect to the *Zang Fu*. They are indicated in any chronic problem.

Lower *He* Sea points are used only for the yang channels. They enhance the effect of any yang Channel problem by assisting the Upper Arm Yang channel.

☯ *Zhang Ying Qing Quan Xi Xue Wei Fang Fa* – Zhang's Holographic Point Location Method

Quan Xi, or Holographic image is a method that allows us the flexibility in selecting acupuncture points even though a point is not traditionally indicated for a particular disease. For example, Pc 7 is typically not indicated for neck pain or headache, but when we use the concept of holographic image, and apply it to the radial bone in the forearm, we can readily use Pc 7 for headaches (particularly *Jue Yin* type) as well as neck pain.

Below: Zhang's 12 points method of holographic acupuncture applied on the Second Metacarpal Bone:

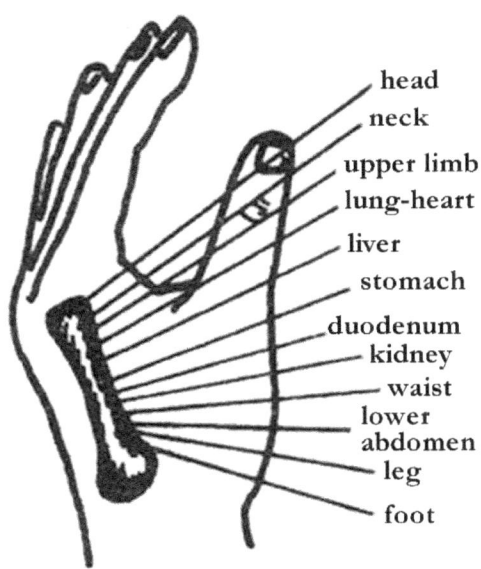

The method we discuss here derives from the work of Dr. Zhang Yingqing of Shandong University, *but I have experimented and added my own thinking here, and applied it into the clinic.*

Dr. Zhang is the director of the ECIWO (Embryo Containing the Information of the Whole Organism) Institute, is the founder of ECIWO Biology, and nationally recognized in China for his outstanding contribution. Based on observation and experiments, Dr. Zhang found that ECIWO is the new unitive unit of structure and function of organism, and finally gave a new view of entire organism—ECIWO theory. Dr.Zhang said that ECIWOs are the specialized embryos that compose the organism and are in some developing stages. .

ECIWO acupuncture or Bio-holographic diagnosis and therapy was founded in 1973 by Dr. Zhang.

ECIWO acupuncture is a medical technique applying ECIWO concepts to acupuncture. ECIWO diagnosis mainly includes diagnosis by electroeciwograph for diagnosis and ECIWO pressure pain (known as "*Ashi*" to us acupuncturists) acupoints diagnosis. ECIWO therapy mainly includes treating by ECIWO instrument for treatment and ECIWO acupuncture and massage. ECIWO acupuncture has been applied in treating 1,000,000 cases with more than 200 kinds of disease. The average effect rate is more than 90%. Surprising effect is often met. ECIWO acupuncture was verified and applied by doctors of more than 30 countries and regions.

The theory of ECIWO acupuncture is profound while the method is simple and highly effective.

ECIWO acupuncture boasts to treat many diseases, including, cerebral thrombosis, cerebral hemorrhage, cerebral hemiplegia, traumatic amputation, cerebral arteriosclerosis, hypertension, concussion of brain, polyneuritis, vascular headache, vertigo, insomnia, lethargy, facial paralysis, facial spasm, tachycardia, hepatitis, gastrospasm, gastroptosis, gastric ulcer, anorexia, tracheitis, cholecystitis, constipation, cirrhosis, dysentery, enuresis, arthritis, scapulohumeral periarthritis, protrusion of intervertebral disc, chronic appendicitis, menopausal syndrome, erosion of cervix, dysmenorrhea, amenorrhea, mastitis, otitis media, pharyngitis, tonsillitis, toothache, rhinitis, conjunctivitis, hemorrhoids, urticaria, orchitis, operative syndrome, infantile diarrhea, neurosis, diabetes, coronary heart disease, renal colic, hyperplasia of prostate, infantile procrastinate pneumonia, infantile procrastinate diarrhea, infantile intestinal obstruction, infantile hyperthermia convulsions, infantile anorexia, abnormal fetal position, rheumatoid disease, cervical spondylopathy, sprain, sports injury, soft tissue injury, intercostal neuralgia, acute cholecystitis, acute gastroenteritis, acute intestinal obstruction, biliary ascariasis, duodenal bulbar inflammation, anal fissures, gastric ulcer, duodenal ulcer, rheumatoid arthritis, rheumatic arthritis, nerve deafness, motion sickness, myopia, acute lower limb phlebitis; pain caused by cancer as breast cancer, esophagus cancer, carcinoma of stomach, liver cancer, lung cancer, intestinal cancer, cancer of pancreas, carcinoma of uterine cervix.

ECIWO Acupuncture has been involved in clinical control studies in China, that show the curative effect of ECIWO therapy is higher than that of Western modern and TCM in treating many kinds of disease.

Zhang Yingqing's theory is that the whole body is projected on all composing parts, as in a holographic system. Zhang Yingqing assessed that the body may be treated with the 2nd metacarpal bone. When we superimpose the normally used anatomical chart onto any of the bones of the body, we can treat the body through selected areas.

I admire Dr. Zhang's work and believe it to be of enormous value in acupuncture, however, I see that Dr. Zhang's work may have a limitation on the traditional acupuncture model. In essence, it is in my opinion, that he forgot the importance of Yin and Yang and that the direction of the treatment points may be flipped, and superimposed vertically, horizontally and in other directions on various body parts, and that in acupuncture proper, we do not only use the bones for treatment, but rather the channels. So in essence, instead of one holograph overlayed on a bone, we should overlay the holograph on the 12 regular channels and in-between the channels. This, in essence, would be a more powerful usage of acupuncture and contribute to the explanation, rational, and flexibility in explaining acupuncture points.

We can then flip the above Holographic Image to obtain more possible locations to treat. For example, area distal to the elbow crease corresponding to the foot will also treat the head.

Quan Xi also makes complete use of the *Zang Xiang* (functions of the organs). If internal organs are involved, we may use points associated with the Yin/Yang organs in the Holographic Image. For example, middle region of the forearm will treat stomach/spleen disorders.

Quan Xi should take into account the *Jing-luo* (Channels and collaterals system). I propose that the Holographic Images correspond to the 12 or 17 major areas of the body on a particular channel, as in the illustration on page 108. For example, for *Yang Ming* headache, we may treat with *Jue Yin* points in the wrist, or Spleen points at the ankle, Lung point in the elbow crease.

Below: Zhang's latest method of holographic acupuncture:

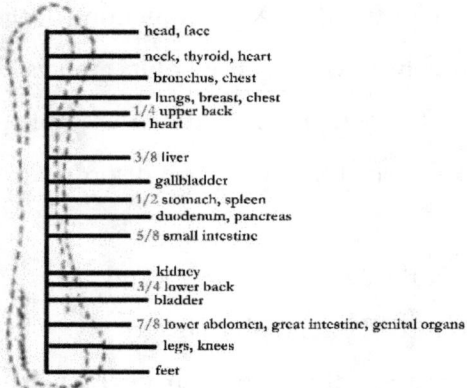

- head, face
- neck, thyroid, heart
- bronchus, chest
- lungs, breast, chest
- 1/4 upper back
- heart
- 3/8 liver
- gallbladder
- 1/2 stomach, spleen
- duodenum, pancreas
- 5/8 small intestine
- kidney
- 3/4 lower back
- bladder
- 7/8 lower abdomen, great intestine, genital organs
- legs, knees
- feet

Master Tung's Essential Points

Finger Points (11.00 position)

Fu Ke 婦科 – Gynecology

Location
On the F line of the proximal segment of the dorsal thumb,
2 points proportionally equidistant between the epicondyles of the
proximal segment of the thumb.

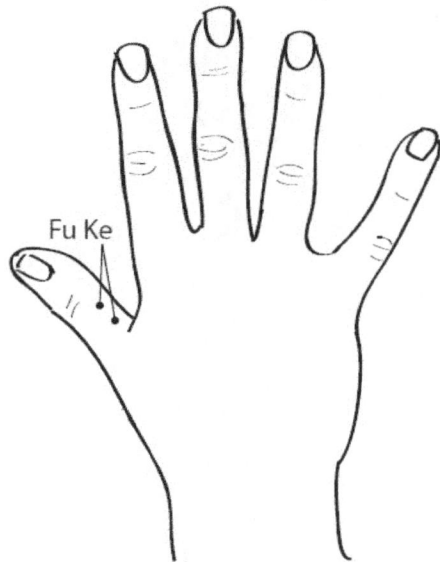

Indications
Vaginitis, ovarian cysts, uterine inflammation, uterine pain, fibroid
tumors, abdominal bloating, irregular menstruation, menstrual
cramps, excessive or scanty menstruation, infertility.

Wu Hu 五虎 – Five Tigers

Location
On the A line of the thumb, along the radial aspect of the proximal segment of the palmar thumb, the 5 points are proportionately equidistant between the epicondyles. Wu Hu 1 is the most distal.

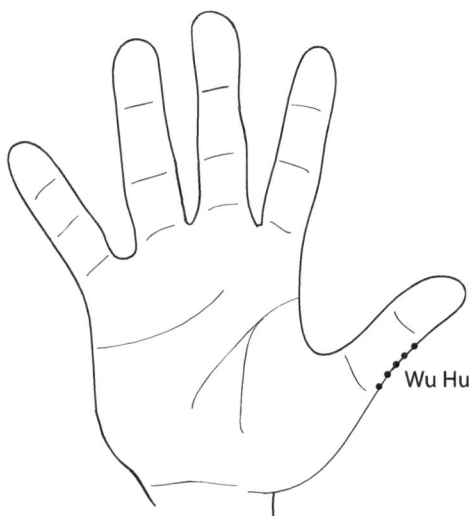

Indications
To treat the whole body wind cold damp Bi syndrome, arthritis, joint pain and swelling.

Wu Hu 1 treats pain of the fingers.
Wu Hu 2 treats pain of the hand/palm.
Wu Hu 3 treats pain of the toes or used as Dao Ma Zhen w/ others
Wu Hu 4 treats pain of the dorsal foot.
Wu Hu 5 treats pain of the heel or plantar region.

Hand Points (22.00 position)

Ling Gu 靈骨– Adroit/Spiritual Bone; Da Bai 大白– Big White

Location
Ling Gu is located at the junction of the first and second metacarpal bones on the LI channel. Da Bai is located at LI 3.

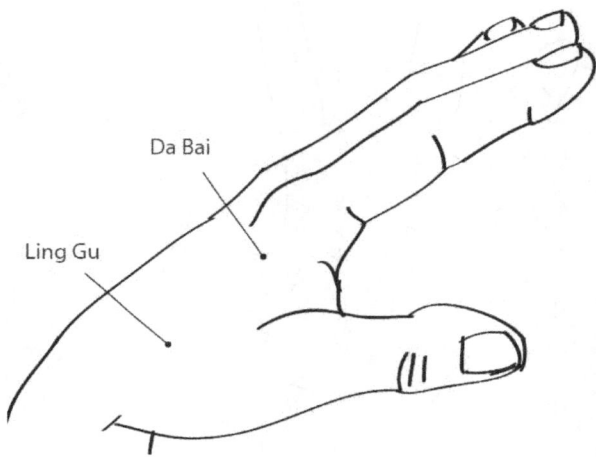

Indications
In general, any Yang Ming channel problems, leg pain and weakness, sciatica, low back pain, hemiplegia, foot pain, and arm pain. These are the most powerful points in Tung's Acupuncture and the most versatile points to move Qi and Blood. When combined with another point or points along an affected channel, Ling Gu and Da Bai can treat almost any disease. Please refer to the following chart to see possible combinations. In essence, Ling Gu and Dai are the sum of Master Tung's genius.

Ling Gu, Da Bai Diseased Area:	Add Guiding Point
Head	Lu 7
Face	LI 3
Eyes	Liv 2
Mouth	St 44
Throat	SJ 2
Neck	GB 39
Back of Neck	UB 65
Shoulders	Sp 9
Scapula	Liv 6
Upper Back	Liv 6
Lower Back	UB 40
Chest	Pc 6
Abdomen	St 36
Lower Abdomen	St 36
Groin	Liv 3
Hypochondrium	GB 34
Anus	Du 26
Gynecological	Sp 6
Vessels	Lu 9
Bones	Shen Guan
Zang	Sp 9
Fu	St 36
Qi	Pc 6
Blood	Sp 10
Sinews	GB 34
Marrow	GB 39
Upper Jiao	Yin Tang
Middle Jiao	Ren 12
Lower Jiao	Ren 6
Pain in Channels	Channel Xi Cleft

Upper Arm Points Reference
(44. Position)

Jian Zhong 肩中 – Shoulder Center

Location:
On the LI Channel, at the center of the deltoid muscle, 2.5 cun distal
to LI 15.

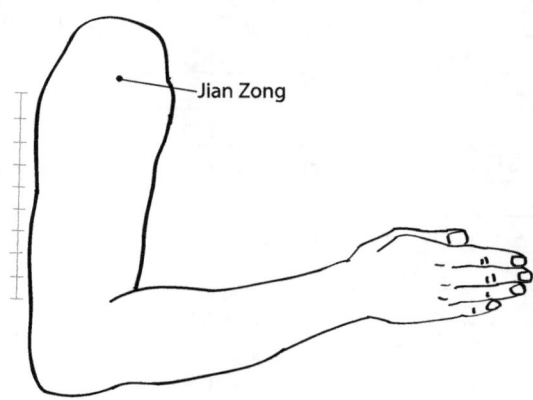

Indications: knee pain, skin disease, polio, stroke, palpitations,
arteriosclerosis, nose bleed, sinusitis, neck pain, headache,
Shoulder Pain, Hemiplegia, Hemiparesis, Epistaxis, Frozen Shoulder,
Ankle Pain, Pain of the Lower leg, Thigh Pain

**Comments: Palpate deeply for the upper epicondyle of the
humerus**

Dorsum and Side of the Foot Points (66.00 position)

Zu Wu Hu 足五虎 1- 5/ Foot Five Tigers

Location
These points are discovered by Robert Chu. These are 5 points equidistant found at the proximal segment of the big toes distal to Sp 2 on the junction of the red and white skin.

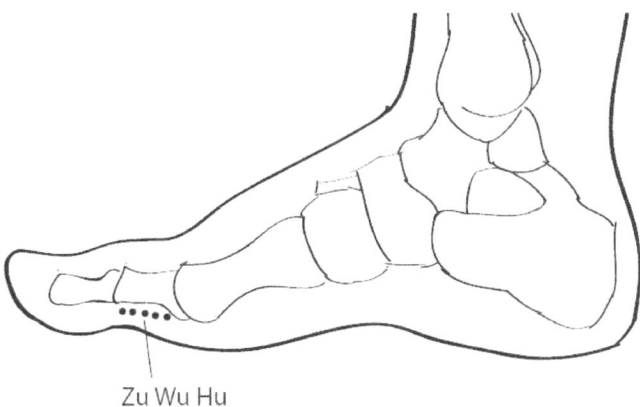

Zu Wu Hu

Indications
Zu Wu Hu 1 is indicated for finger pain.

Zu Wu Hu 2 is indicated in hand pain.

Zu Wu Hu 3 is indicated in toe pain or is used to assist other Zu Wu Hu points.

Zu Wu Hu 4 is indicated in the top of the foot pain.

Zu Wu Hu 5 is indicated in plantar or heel pain.

Huo Ying 火硬– Fire Hard; Huo Zhu 火主– Fire Ruler

Location
Huo Ying is found 0.5 cun posterior to Liv 2; Huo Zhu is located just distal to the junction of the 1st and 2nd metatarsal bones.

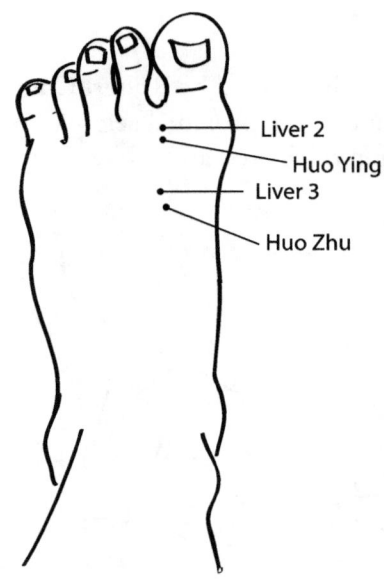

Indications
Palpitations, vertigo, heart weakness, uterine inflammation, fibroid tumors, headaches due to heart disease, liver yang rising, TMJ, groin pain, prostatitis.

Men Jin 門 金 – Gate of Gold

Location

Men Jin is located at St 43, just distal to the junction of the second and third metatarsal bones.

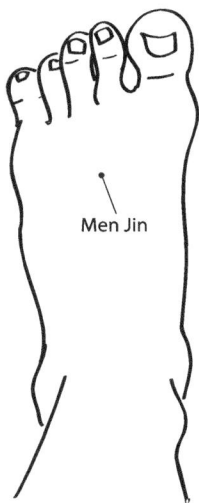

Indications: Diarrhea, gas and bloating, and digestive problems, Appendicitis, Dysmenorrhea, Abdominal Pain, Middle finger pain, Instep Pain, Abdominal distention, Thigh Pain

Mu Dou 木斗– Wood Combat; Mu Liu木留 – Wood Remains

Location
Mu Dou is located 0.5 cun from web margin between 3rd and 4th metatarsal bones. Mu Liu is anterior to the junction of the 3rd and 4th metatarsal bones.

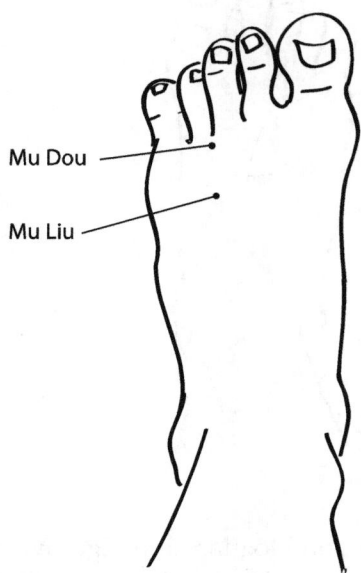

Mu Dou

Mu Liu

Indication
Splenomegaly, indigestion, liver disease, fatigue, polio, St/GB problems. Also treats whole body numbness due to poor circulation, finger pain, stiff neck and shoulder blade pain.

Lower Leg Points (77 position)

Qi Hu 七 虎 – Seven Tigers

Location: 3 points, the first is 2 cun above UB 60, the 2nd point is 2 cun above the first, the 3rd point is 2 cun above the 2nd.

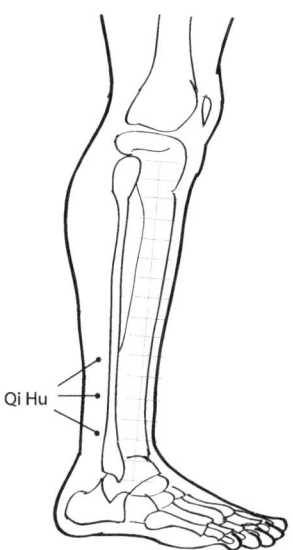

Indications:

Neck pain, Shoulder pain, clavicle pain, Pneumonia,

Yi Chong 一 重 – First Layer; Er Chong 二重 – Second Layer; San Chong 三重 – Third Layer

Location
Yi Chong is at GB 39; Er Chong is 2 cun above Yi Chong; San Chong is 2 cun above Er Chong. Collectively, they are known as San Chong as a Hui Ma set.

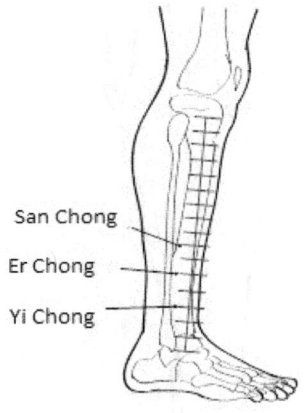

San Chong
Er Chong
Yi Chong

Indications

Goiter, exopthalmous, Bell's palsy, migraine headaches, neck pain, thyroid tumor, generally used for hyperthyroidism and/or goiter.

Tian Huang 天 皇– Heaven Emperor
Shen Guan 腎關, also known as Tian Huang Fu 天皇附
Di Huang 地皇 – Earth Emperor
Ren Huang 人皇 – Human Emperor

Location: Tian Huang point is Sp 9, it is found on the Spleen channel below the medial condyle of tibia bone, along the tibial border.

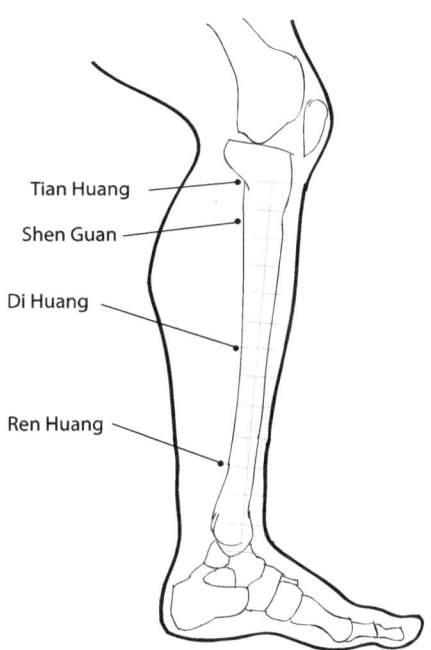

Indications: Hyperacidity of the Stomach, nephritis, diabetes, proteinurea, frequent urination, prostatitis, heart disease, vertigo, insomnia, high blood pressure, neck pain, shoulder pain, treats Sp, K, Liver channels, Atherosclerosis, Anemia, Abdominal pain, Hemorrhoids, Endocarditis, Myocardial infarction, Pericarditis, Hypotension, Adrenal gland disorders, Obesity, Forearm Pain, Upper Arm Pain

Combine With: Di Huang and Ren Huang

Comments: For more Spleen disorders

Shen Guan 腎關, also known as Tian Huang Fu 天皇附 – Kidney Gate, Heaven Emperor Appendage

Location: Shen Guan point is found 1.5 cun below Sp 9.

Indications: Asthma, SOB, prostatitis, acid reflux, astigmatism, anemia, epilepsy, mental disease, vertigo, all diseases due to Kidney Qi deficiency including sciatica, lower back pain, headaches, shoulder pain, hip pain, Shoulder Pain, Wrist Pain, Lateral Elbow pain, Hemorrhoids, Epilepsy, Pain in the supraorbital region, Dizziness, Endocarditis, Hypertension, Chronic pulmonary heart disease, Pericarditis, Myocarditis, Obesity

Combine With: Di Huang, Ren Huang
Comments: Can be used singly for shoulder pain.

Di Huang 地皇 – Earth Emperor

Location: Di Huang point is found on the Spleen Channel, 7 cun above the tip of the medial malleolus. According to Li Guo Zhen, this point is found 3.5 cun above the point 77.21 Ren Huang – Human Emperor

Indications: Nephritis, lower leg edema, diabetes, gonorrhea, impotence, premature ejaculation, proteinurea, hematurea, fibroid tumors, irregular menses, lower back pain due to Kidney Qi deficiency, Atherosclerosis, Anemia, Spermatorrhea, Essential hypertension, Endometriosis, Hypotension, Adrenal gland disorders, Obesity, Forearm Pain

Combine With: Shen Guan, Ren Huang

Comments: Together, these are the famous **Xia San Huang** points, the "Lower Three Emperors"

Ren Huang 人皇 – Human Emperor

Location: Ren Huang is on the Spleen Channel, this point is found 3 cun above the tip of the medial malleolus, along the tibial border. This point is located at Sp 6. According to other sources, this point is 3.5 cun superior to the tip of the medial malleolus. Some have said that the point is 3 cun above the medial malleolus.

Indications: Gonorrhea, impotence, premature ejaculation, lumbago, cervicalgia, vertigo, numb hands, diabetes, blood in urine, nephritis, kidney Qi deficiency, Atherosclerosis, Anemia, Upper Back Pain, Upper Back Stiffness, Wrist Pain, Dizziness, Spermatorrhea, Cystitis, Essential hypertension, Numbness and pain of the upper extremities, Hypotension, Adrenal gland disorders, Obesity, Forearm Pain

Combine With: Shen Guan, Di Huang
Comments: Together, these are the famous **Xia San Huang** points, the "Lower Three Emperors"

Ce San Li 側三里– Side of Three Miles - 133
Ce Xia San Li 側下三里– Along Side Below San Li - 134

Location
Ce San Li is level with St 36, 0.5 cun lateral; Ce Xia San Li is 2 cun below Ce San Li.

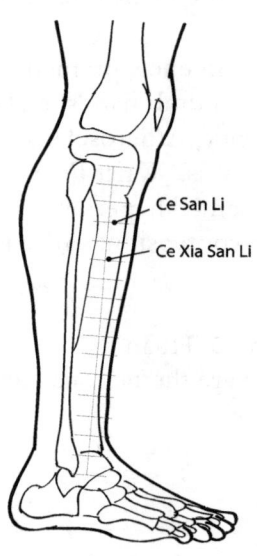

Indications
All problems along the Yang Ming and Shao Yang channels including migraine headache, toothaches, trigeminal neuralgia pain, wrist pain, finger stiffness, Otitis media, and TMJ

Thigh Points (88.00 position)

Si Ma Zhong 駟馬中 Chariot Horses Middle Si Ma Shang 駟馬上;– Chariot Horses Upper; Si Ma Xia 駟馬下 – Chariot Horses Lower Three Chariot Horses – Chariot Middle, Upper, and Lower; Collectively known as Si Ma San

Location

Si Ma Zhong is found 4 fingerbreadths anterior to GB 31, Si Ma Shang is 2 cun superior, Si Ma Xia is 2 cun inferior.

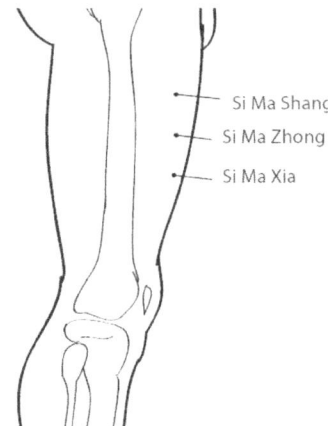

Indications

These are Master Tung's best points to treat Lung Channel conditions, including allergies, sinus and skin conditions including eczema and psoriasis, and also chest pain, and palpitations

Zhong Jiu Li 中九里– Center Nine Miles; Shang Jiu Li 上九里 – Upper Nine Miles; Xia Jiu Li 下九里 – Lower Nine Miles; Collectively known as "San Jiu Li"

Location
Zhong Jiu Li is located at GB 31; Shang Jiu Li is 1.5 cun anterior, Xia Jiu Li is 1.5 cun posterior to Zhong Jiu Li.

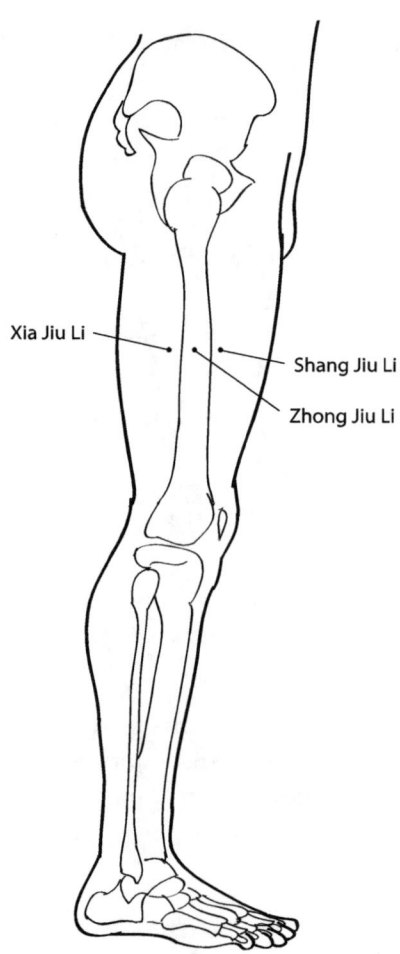

Indications
Back pain, lower back pain, disc pain, stroke, Bell's palsy, neck pain, vertigo, eyeball fullness, hand numbness, arm numbness, leg pain, weakness in the legs, migraine headache, rashes, hives, and tinnitis.

Head and Face Points
(1010.00 position)

Bi Yi 鼻翼一 Nasal wing

Location: This point is located at the superior depression of ala nasi. This is located where most women would place their nose ring.

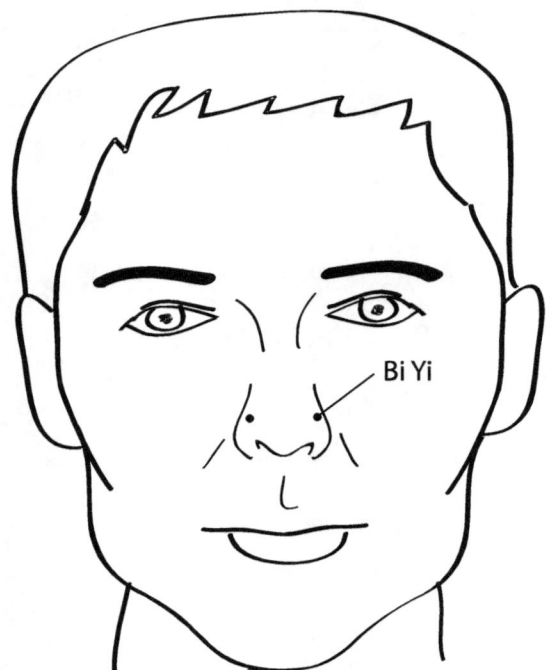

Indications: Fatigue, pain due to Qi related conditions, headache, sore throat, migraines.

Some Explanation

In this section, I will discuss the logic presented in this book for choosing classical acupuncture points derived from the channel pathways and imaging and give some insights into the Master Tung's points. I am not trying to recreate a treatment formulary here, but rather, show the logic that goes into my other works, **Master Tung's Acupuncture for Pain**, and **Master Tung's Acupuncture for Internal Medicine Disorders**. Once the general idea is understood, you will have a complete roadmap for using the Master Tung system in your clinic immediately. For those who would like to learn more in-depth about creating prescriptions, and more of Master Tung's points, they should refer to my work, **The Best of Master Tung's Acupuncture**. The Appendix in this book does have some sample treatments for some common ailments to start from.

Treating Neck and Shoulder and Throat Pain

Acupuncture is a targeting system. Like GPS, if we know the longitude and latitude, you will have a destination. In Acupuncture, once we know the channels, and can determine which ones we select to treat a problem, we then use an imaging system. The combination of channel, plus imaging, will allow us to treat most problems instantly.

In treating neck pain, we have to identify first, where is the pain?

Let's say the pain in in the GB area of the neck, between the points GB 20 and GB 21. Well, on the simplest level, we could needle that same point on the opposite side using our understanding of Same Height Imaging.

If we choose to use the legs, like in Foot and Torso Imaging, we would understand that the ankle images the neck region. With this method, we would use the ankle to treat neck problems. We now have the Channel and the Imaging and that equals a point. So using GB 39 would be ideal. And in classical texts like the *Da Cheng*, GB 39 is considered the best point to treat neck pain.

As TCM trained acupuncturists, we know that GB 39 *Xuanzhong*/Suspended Bell is located on the lateral aspect of the lower leg, 3 cun above the tip of the external malleolus, on the anterior border of the fibula.

Indeed, GB 39, besides being the influential point of marrow, is used in cases of all neck issues, neck stiffness, arthritis of the neck, neck strain, neck sprain, whiplash, and headaches.

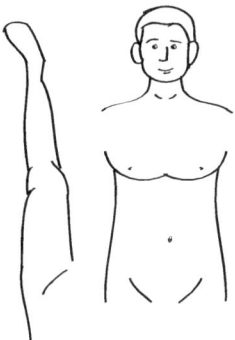

If the problem were pain in the neck in the UB Channel area, we could again use the above imaging and think which point corresponds to the neck region along the UB Channel. Using Foot and Torso Imaging, we know that the ankle images the neck region, and would then consider a point on the ankle on the UB channel to treat the neck pain. Again, we have the channel and the imaging, so we have a point. A good point then would be to use UB 60.

UB 60, known as *Kun Lun*, referring to the *Kun Lun* mountains, is located on the foot, behind the external malleolus, in the depression between the tip of the external malleolus and tendo-calcaneus. It is often used for lumbar pain, swelling and pain of the heel, difficult labor, headache, neck stiffness, dizziness, epistaxis, and infantile convulsions. TCM simply lists these indications as "headache" and neck "stiffness", but because we know that it is on the Urinary Bladder channel, it is for Tai Yang type headaches and Tai Yang neck pain.

If we use the above two examples of GB and UB channel neck pain and use the same logic using Master Tung's points, we can clearly see why Master Tung taught the San Chong Hui Ma set and the Qi Hu Hui Ma sets as go to points for neck and shoulder pain. Both will treat neck and shoulder pain on their respective channels.

As we recall, San Chong Hui Ma set is made up of three points, the first is Yi Chong, which is at GB 39. The second point, Er Chong is 2 cun above Yi Chong. San Chong, the third point is 2 cun above Er Chong. Collectively, they are known as the San Chong Hui Ma set. If we look at the imaging, they are the ankle points moving down to the side of the calf muscle. This would indicate, that the points were not only good for neck pain, but for shoulder pain, and upper back pain.

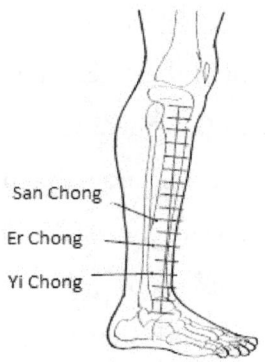

The Qi Hu Hui Ma set, would address then, neck, shoulder pain and upper back pain more on the Urinary Bladder channel. We still use the same imaging of the leg and torso, but this time we are more on the UB channel. The image and the channel leads to our selection of points.

Qi Hu or Seven Tigers is a set of three points with the first located 2 cun above UB 60; the second point is 2 cun above the first; and the third point is 2 cun above the 2nd.

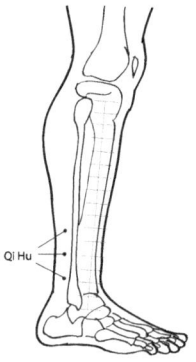

Of course, we can address neck pain, or even throat pain very simply in this method. Assuming throat or neck pain would be at the St 9 or LI 18 area, we can safely choose St 41 to treat this. St 41, or Jie Xie Stream Divide is at the junction of the dorsum of the foot and the lower leg, in the depression at the midpoint of the transverse crease of the ankle between the tendons m. extensor hallucis longus and digitorum longus. Classical Acupuncture, however, does acknowledge this as a "*Jing* River

Point" and it is used to address all issues of the lungs that relate to cough and sore throat. Although the TCM point indication for St 41 does not say it will treat neck or throat pain, we understand that this is under imaging and channel a point that will treat these problems. If there were pain extending down the throat to the clavicle, we can simply palpate for *Ashi* point reaction areas between St 41 and St 40.

This is also an advantage of why our Master Tung's Acupuncture is more fun and creative to use in the clinic.

Knee Pain

Knee pain is commonly seen in the clinic and causes might be due to Arthralgia (joint pain) of lower leg or knee, Knee joint pain. Patellofemoral syndrome, Meniscus partial tear, and a host of other reasons. If it doesn't require surgery, most likely, acupuncture can help this. Often, patients play sports like basketball, snowboarding, or football, and wind up with knee pain of sorts. Again, we can use Master Tung's imaging and channel methods to aid us.

The imaging method of the Hand and Foot, are probably best suited for this problem. The idea is to have the elbow treat the knees. Hand and Foot Imaging, as we recall, is the elbow corresponds to the knee.

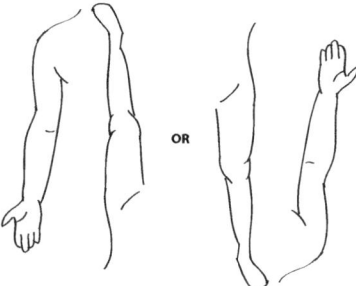

Since we have imaging, all we need now is the channel involved. Usually knee pain is either the medial, lateral, through the patella, or the back of the knee. With knowledge of our channels pathways, we can easily use the Same Channel Name method for choosing the points.

Tong Ming Jing Fang Fa or the Hand and Foot Same Channels Name Method is when we exploit the same channel name relationship, for example, both the Lung and Spleen are Tai Yin; therefore use the Lung to treat the Spleen. Since the Yang Ming channel is composed of the Large Intestine and Stomach Channels, use them to treat each other.

As we recall, this breaks down as:

Troubled Channel	Treat with this channel
Lung	Spleen
Large Intestine	Stomach
Stomach	Large Intestine
Spleen	Lung

Heart	Kidney
Small Intestine	Urinary Bladder
Urinary Bladder	Small Intestine
Kidney	Heart
Pericardium	Liver
San Jiao	Gall Bladder
Gall Bladder	San Jiao
Liver	Pericardium

So if knee pain is medial, we would use the Lu 5 point to treat the knee pain, as it would most likely be Leg Tai Yin Spleen Channel involved.

If knee pain were around St 35 or St 36, we would then choose LI 11 to treat the pain.

If it were the back of the knee that was pained, we could try Lu 5, as we recall, there is the branching relationship of each channel. In that case, Tai Yin and Tai Yang treat each other and the Lu 5 could certainly treat UB 40 Knee pain.

If the knee pain were around the Jue Yin channel, we could treat using Master Tung's special points, Huo Ying 火硬– Fire Hard; Huo Zhu 火主– Fire Ruler. Huo Ying is found 0.5 cun posterior to Liv

2; Huo Zhu is located just distal to the junction of the 1st and 2nd
metatarsal bones.

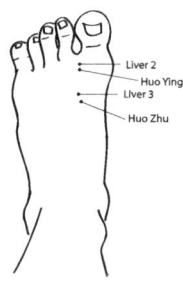

These points treat Knee Pain miraculously. If we think of the logic
of why these points work, we can see that they're very close to the
Ying Spring and *Shu* Stream points of the Liver Channel. *Ying* Spring
points are indicated in inflammation, whereas *Shu* Stream points are
indicated in joint pain. Since knees are joints, it makes sense that if
there is pain on the knees, there is probably inflammation, so using
points that have the properties of treating inflammation in the joints
are good.

Hangovers, Fatigue, Headaches, and "Chemobrain"

Often, patients come to my clinic for different ailments. Perhaps
they partied too much, went to a bar, went to meet ladies, got drunk.
Or they've just had a bad night, feeling fatigue, and can't sleep.
Sometimes they have headaches or suffer from migraines. Some of
my patients have the phenomenon known as "chemobrain" in
oncology circles, it's when a patient is treated with chemotherapy or
radiation therapy, and the patient becomes forgetful. They can't

remember where they put their keys, wallet, phone, or appointments. They suffer from nausea and vomiting, and can't keep any food in. Probably some of that is from worry, toxins, and fatigue. What I do for them is use a combination of points that I have found particularly effective for them. I combine the Master Tung's *Bi Yi*, with *Huo Ying* and *Huo Zhu*. I do plan on writing more about oncology treatment of side effects in another future work.

Bi Yi is a special point. These days, it's become a trend, where many women find it fashionable to have their noses pierced and wear a nose ring. *Bi Yi* is at the end of the nasal labial groove, at the superior depression of *ala nasi*. As it is right on the ala nasi of the nose, hence the name, *Bi Yi* "Nasal Wing".

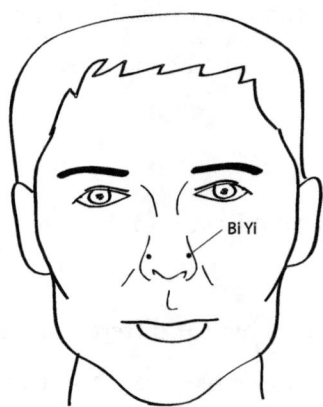

Bi Yi is used for conditions of fatigue, pain due to Qi related conditions, headache, sore throat, and migraines. As this point is on the nose, and we know same height imaging method, we know that it will also treat occipital headache.

Huo Ying and *Huo Zhu* have already been discussed before, but I will point out that with the relationship of the channels, the Liver Channel will treat the Gall Bladder, Liver collateral, and Stomach channels, therefore covering most of your bases for headache and fatigue with this set of points.

Now in these few sentences, I believe many are starting to understand the depth and flexibility and power in Tung's points. As this is a Primer, and not an exhaustive text to explore all treatment possibilities, I leave you with this to work out. My other works will give you a more well-rounded picture of the Master Tung Acupuncture system.

Of course, I still give seminars nationally and internationally to explain the Master Tung system in person, as acupuncture is a physical medicine and requires kinesthetic touch to experience.

Dr. Chu's 10 Needle Protocol

For beginners, it's great to use my "Dr. Chu 10 Needle Protocol" Rx as a basic template in treating all types of chronic diseases. It is a good example using Tung's acupuncture and the principle of channel circuits, as well as using Master Tung's preference for treating the Liver, Gallbladder, Stomach, and Spleen channels for chronic conditions.

We treat the Spleen and Stomach based on Li Dong Yuan's "Treatise of the Spleen and Stomach". Spleen and Stomach is like the alternator of the car - it charges the battery (Kidneys). You could have a fresh car battery that will say it can last 5 years, but without the alternator, your car battery would drain in a day or so. So without treating the Spleen and Stomach properly, your entire system would fall apart. That is why I treat the Spleen and Stomach in chronic disease and not the Kidneys.

Modern living is time bound and stressful, and you read everything with your eyes, and have to make quick decisions all the time - this is why I treat the wood elements - the Liver and Gallbladder.

The whole idea is to have a basic template or roadmap to treat patients and then modify accordingly with additional points if necessary.

Huo Ying, Huo Zhu	*Xia San Huang*
Liv 6	St 36, 37
GB 34, 39	

The standard points of Liv 6, GB 34 and GB 39, St 36, and St 37 are common and all acupuncturists know them. *Huo Ying* and *Huo Zhu* are famous points of Master Tung as are the *Xia San Huang* points.

It is said in Chinese Medicine Classics that the Gallbladder is responsible for determination and flexibility, so it is only natural that I chose to use the points GB 34, as it is the Influential point of tendons, and GB 39, as it is the influential point of marrow. Affecting the tendons allows you to relax. Affecting the marrow also helps you relax as it relaxes the mind, brain, and cerebral spinal fluid.

Liv 6 is chosen, as it is the Xi Cleft point of the Liver, and it is used in acute cases of irritability, anger, frustration, a common occurrence in time bound society. Pain in the hypochondrium, abdominal distention and pain, diarrhea are also indications for Liv 6. We should remember that Xi-Cleft points are where Qi of the channels is deeply converged. *Ashi* reaction upon palpation of the Xi Cleft points, show pathogens have entered deeply into the *Zang Fu*. *Xi* Cleft points are often used for acute, painful symptoms, inflammation, and protracted diseases of the particular channel affected. Finally, *Xi* Cleft points are used for hemostatic effect.

St 36 is one of the most common points used in all acupuncture. It is known as the command point of the abdomen and chest, the He Sea point of the Stomach channel, the Sea of Water and Grain, and is used for "tonifying" Qi and Blood, strengthens the Spleen and Stomach, strengthens the body, fortifies Wei qi, raises Yang, calms the Shen, and stops pain. When coupled with St 37, the lower He Sea point of the Large Intestine, it serves to drain downward, detox, move the bowels, clear heat, and who doesn't feel better when they have a bowel movement? St 37 is commonly indicated for acute appendicitis, abdominal pain, borborygmus, constipation, diarrhea, muscular atrophy, weakness, and for numbness and pain of the lower extremities. In our society, I see many patients who lack a regularity of bowel movements. Sigmund Freud would refer to these patients as *"anal retentive"*.

Huo Ying is found 0.5 cun posterior to Liv 2; *Huo Zhu* is located just distal to the junction of the 1st and 2nd metatarsal bones.

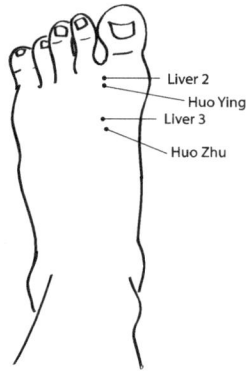

Since these are on the Liver Channel and are basically the *Ying* Spring and *Shu* Stream points, they can treat all types of inflammation and joint pain. *Shu* Stream points are also indicated to moving things along quickly to stop Liver Qi Stagnation, a problem in our society, which leads to anger issues, insomnia, depression, and a host of internal medicine diseases like hypertension, high cholesterol, metabolic syndrome, and the like.

The other *Hui Ma* set of points is the famous *Xia San Huang* combination. They consist of the points, *Shen Guan* 腎關, also known as *Tian Huang Fu* 天皇附 – Kidney Gate, Heaven Emperor Appendage, *Di Huang* 地皇 – Earth Emperor, and *Ren Huang* 人皇 – Human Emperor.

Shen Guan point is found 1.5 cun below Sp 9. *Di Huang* point is found on the Spleen Channel, 7 cun above the tip of the medial malleolus, along the border of the tibia. According to Lee Kuo-

chen, this point is found 3.5 cun above the point 77.21 *Ren Huang* –
Human Emperor. *Ren Huang* is on the Spleen Channel, this point
is found 3 cun above the tip of the medial malleolus, along the
tibial border. This point is located at the common location of Sp 6.
According to other sources, this point is 3.5 cun superior to the tip
of the medial malleolus. Dr. Wang Chuan-min has said this point is 3
cun above the medial malleolus.

Shen Guan can be used singly for shoulder pain, asthma, or prostate
issues. *Di Huang* is used in combination with *Shen Guan* and *Ren
Huang*, but can be used singly for midback pain. *Ren Huang* is used
for a host of gynecological and reproductive problems, including
Gonorrhea, impotence, premature ejaculation, anemia, and
Spermatorrhea.

However, the synergistic functions of the famous **Xia San Huang**,
the "Lower Three Emperors", include most of the modern diseases
mentioned before including hypertension, high cholesterol, metabolic
syndrome, diabetes, hypothyroidism, and gallbladder disease.

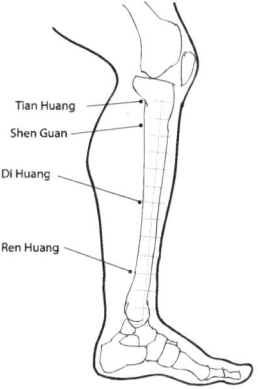

If Li Dong Yuan lived in modern times, he would probably agree with me that we live in the age of "Liver, Gall Bladder, Spleen and Stomach" diseases.

An Interview with Robert Chu, PhD, LAc, QME, about ITARA, by Jack Chang

Robert Chu, L.Ac., QME, PhD, has been practicing the Martial and Chinese healing arts since childhood and specializes in Master Tung Acupuncture and Optimal Acupuncture methods for treating pain, neuromusculoskeletal disorders, and internal medicine problems. He founded, in mid 2005, ITARA (International Tung's Acupuncture Research Association), a non-political organization devoted to the preservation, standardization, education, and research of Tung's Acupuncture, offering classes for the spread and advancement of Tung's Acupuncture for clinical efficacy. He has been teaching internationally throughout the United States, Europe and Canada at various Chinese Medicine symposiums, including CSOMA, AAOM, AOM Alliance, COMS, and other functions as an exciting and dynamic speaker.

In July of 2004, Dr. Chu was selected as the Acupuncturist to Olympic athletes at the Olympic Trials held in Sacramento, CA.

Jack Chang is a licensed Acupuncturist in San Francisco, CA.. He has been studying martial arts since 1995. He is also a disciple of Robert Chu studying martial arts and acupuncture. He is certified in Tui Na Massage. He has been practicing bodywork and qi gong healing since 2002, specializing in upper back pain and repetitive work related injuries.

Jack Chang (JC): What does ITARA stand for?

Robert Chu (RC): ITARA was founded in 2004, and our name is an acronym that stands for **International Tung's Acupuncture Research Association**. The acronym is a play on the bodhisattva, Tara, a being that will help others cross over to wisdom and compassion for all sentient beings. I hope that every healthcare practitioner can find the Tara within them.

JC: What inspired you to create ITARA?

RC: I have a vision to share with all acupuncturists – to form a non-political atmosphere of sharing Master Tung's Acupuncture. I don't think people study Tung's Acupuncture to become mini-clones of Master Tung, but rather, to become clinically effective and efficient. Right now in Taiwan and in the USA, people are branching off and saying they study this branch or that branch of the Tung's Acupuncture, but this is wrong. They shouldn't be trying to propagate a tradition, but rather strive for clinical efficacy and function. It doesn't matter the lineage, they all have merit. And if some practice certain points and have clinical efficacy, that's what is important. Master Tung's Acupuncture is this great body of work and an example to people practicing acupuncture. Many of his disciples are criticizing each other and there is infighting about market share and money, all stating they have the real deal. Actually, I look at it like the old tale of the elephant and the five blind men – they all say an elephant is like a tree trunk, snake, vine, leaf, wall, but they can't see the elephant!

JC: What are the goals of ITARA?

RC: The goals of ITARA are the preservation, standardization, education, and research of Tung's Acupuncture, and offering practical based classes for the spread and advancement of Tung's Acupuncture. We're wanting to preserve all forms of Tung's Acupuncture, and the interesting variations of it, that work clinically. We can also look to standardize the points – for example the point Da Bai, some say it is LI 3, others say it is ½ cun proximal to LI 3 – everyone argues the fact. If it has clinical merit, then I don't really care, all I care about is if it works. Some in Tung's Acupuncture say the channels are not important, all that is important is Tung's points, but I don't quite agree with that. Of course, the points have a function that is related to the channels in one way of another, or related via correspondence, tissue, imaging, nervous system, or holograph. One cannot say it only works because Tung and the Tung family found these points. Some say that Tung's points should be practiced alone, without the 14 channels points, but we know historically, Master Tung used the regular channel points, then used his family points and finally used the family points in conjunction with the channel points.   Master Tung also has his 5 Zang Channel method, which makes use of his family's approach.

JC: Can you tell me a little about some of the research projects that ITARA is working on?

RC: Well, we're currently working on teaching and seminars throughout the U.S.A., Europe and Canada, creating courses for acupuncturists, doing research into how and why Master Tung's Acupuncture works, and I am discussing projects to do research on Master Tung to prove the efficacy of the Master Tung points, as well as invite other Master Tung practitioners with unique clinical experience to share their experience with us. We don't want to be pigeon holed into one lineage of Master Tung Acupuncture, but really want to understand the merits of all the methods Master Tung passed down. In addition, we have discovered new uses for acupuncture points in TCM as well as the Master Tung system, and flexible methods of applying these points.

For example, we discovered that there are five points on the big toe, just as there are the Wu Hu (Five Tiger) points on the hand. In naming the points, I simply called them "Zu Wu Hu" (Foot Five Tigers) to honor the tradition. Their point location corresponds to the points on the hands and are flexibly applied for finger, hand, toe, top of foot and plantar pain.. We keep discovering other applications and points by flexibly applying Master Tung's Acupuncture principles and concepts, which I think is what every practitioner should do.

JC: Are there any oaths or medical ethics that ITARA members abide by?

RC: Yes, we want to stress that we're clinicians first and not just theoreticians, so I advise my students to "Let function rule over form" and "Let application be your guide". This is more important than blindly following any master, methodology, or rigid adherence to style. If we want to really understand something, it's not important to follow as "Sifu says...", but rather really understand the basic principles and concepts. In this way, we're not caught up in the dogma of what we study. We don't want to be another plain vanilla Master Tung's points course – we want really be an organization that freely disseminates information to our people and applies it clinically. I also want to stress that we respect all teachings, and believe they have their validity.

JC: Who was Master Tung, and where did his acupuncture derive from?

RC: Master Tung Ching-chang was probably the greatest Acupuncturist in the last generation in Taiwan. So great was his fame, that he literally had over 100 patients per day, which he saw in his small clinic. His fame was due to his extreme efficacy with acupuncture needles, and he only used a few per treatment. The Tung family hailed from Pingdu, Shangdong province in China, and were allegedly a family that practiced acupuncture there for generations.

Master Tung arrived in Taiwan after the Communists took over in China in 1949 along with Chiang Kai-shek's Nationalist party and began a successful practice in Taipei, Taiwan. He was an Acupuncturist in Taiwan for 26 years, and throughout that time, he allegedly treated over 400,000 patients, with about a fourth of them treated at no charge. For these humanitarian deeds, Master Tung was decorated with an award of "Representative of Fine People and Fine Deeds" in Taiwan.

As the personal acupuncturist to Taiwan President Chang Kai Shek, his reputation was so great that he was asked to visit Cambodia between 1971 and 1974 to treat Cambodian President Long Nuo, who suffered from hemiplegia due to a stroke.

Master Tung was also decorated by President Chang Kai Shek with a "Certificate of Honor" in the field of Chinese Medicine, which is an amazing accomplishment because initially the Nationalist Party was not responsive to Chinese Medicine, due to the fact that Sun Yat Sen was a Western trained physician.

JC: What's special about Tung's Acupuncture?

RC: Master Tung's Acupuncture is truly a living treasure and storehouse of Chinese Medicine, untouched by modern TCM, and a glimpse into the family systems of Chinese Medicine as taught in previous generations. It is itself a conglomerate of classical acupuncture and pricking methods, flexibly applied, and proven clinically with practical, often with quick and dramatic results. Currently many practitioners of acupuncture may use a lot of needles and needle around the local area. Not so with Master Tung's Acupuncture. For example, if a person has neck pain, a TCM trained acupuncturist would typically needle the neck area. But a Master Tung acupuncturist will apply a few needles to the wrist, ankle, knee, shoulder, hip, or thigh to treat the pain. The advantage is very clear, as you can get feedback immediately from your patient upon insertion. If one needled the neck, for neck pain, one would have to wait until they are removed to get feedback! For the acupuncturist, the flexibility of the method is extremely attractive.

JC: What can you treat with Master Tung's Acupuncture?

RC: Master Tung's acupuncture is painless, quick, efficient and requires only a few treatments if problems are acute. I specializing in pain, women's health, and internal medicine, with a sub-specialty of Cancer Treatment side-effects. A full range of problems are treated, including allergies, anxiety, arthritis, asthma, back pain and sciatica, Bell's Palsy, bronchitis, Carpal Tunnel Syndrome, high blood pressure, colitis, common cold and flu, constipation, diarrhea, ear pain and ringing, eczema and other skin problems, edema, frozen shoulder, GERD, headaches, IBS, impotence, insomnia, laryngitis, menstrual problems, menopause, nausea and vomiting, numbness and neuropathy, pain of all types, PMS, prostate problems, rheumatism, stress, stroke, tennis elbow, TMJ, and Trigeminal Neuralgia with just a few needles. It is almost inconceivable as to the efficacy of this form of acupuncture. In my own daily practice, I am still amazed at the immediate results I see with this system of acupuncture.

JC: Who else practices Tung's Acupuncture in the U.S.A.?

RC: Master Tung's Acupuncture in the USA is practiced by Young Wei-chieh in Rowland Heights, CA, Wang Chuan-min in Chicago, IL, Esther Su of San Jose, CA, Jim Maher of Oklahoma City, OK, and myself. I had the fortune of learning from Esther Su, and did extensive research in this system of acupuncture and practice daily in Pasadena, CA. I also studied with Young Wei-chieh, but am not a disciple or indoor student of his. He was kind to answer what questions I had and I had worked on editing his manual in English, and when I worked as a seminar coordinator and translator for him, for a few seminars in Los Angeles. I later studied with Dr. Wang and learned his classical Master Tung system, and he was instrumental in sending me corrected early texts of Master Tung's Acupuncture.

JC: Are the set of points by Master Tung standardized internationally, and if not do you see it being standardized in the future?

RC: Most of the common points of Tung's Acupuncture are fairly standardized, as we have the written works of Lai Jin Hung, Hu Bing-Quan, Li Guo Zhen, Wang Chuan-min, Liu Yi, Young Wei-chieh. In English, we have works from Palden Carson, Miriam Lee, James Maher, Wang Chuan-min and Young Wei-chieh, most recently. Points like Ling Gu, Si Ma, Tian Huang, Shen Guan are fairly standardized in location and function, but others like Zhong Bai may have different names, different locations, and even different function! What I would like to see is that practitioners of Tung's Acupuncture all meet together and share clinical experiences and discuss civilly the differences and then standardize on the points. Of course, since we're a young organization, something like this is a work in process.

JC: How often do you use Master Tung's points?

RC: I use the Master Tung points daily. Of course, if I don't use the Tung set of points, I use the logic behind the Tung's system to guide my practice in particular with the 12 main channels. For example, a great point to treat *Shao Yang* headache would be GB 43, as the foot images the head and the headache originates in the Gallbladder channel.

JC: What is Optimal Acupuncture and a little taste of an example of Optimal acupuncture?

RC: Optimal Acupuncture © is my own system, combining what I call 6 pillars of knowledge drawing from classical acupuncture, imaging, point properties, chrono-acupuncture, symbolism, and holographs. It is a way to optimize acupuncture taking into consideration time and space. I have clearly described to my students sources and inspirations range from Master Tung, Liu Bing Quan, Peng Jing Shan, Zhang Ying Qing, Huang Li Chun, Paul Nogier, Zhang Xin Shu, Fang Yun Peng, Jiao Shun Fa, Zhu Ming Qing, Chen Chao, Lu Jing Shan and others. As you know, I am also an avid student of the classics *Su Wen, Ling Shu, Nan Jing, Jia Yi Jing, Da Cheng* and *Da Chuan* which are the basis of many of my own insights of Chinese Medicine and the methods I practice in my clinic and share with my students.

An example of Optimal Acupuncture is let's say today is *Ji Si* day – so the Spleen is most active today, we can use the Spleen channel to treat any problem, regardless of what channel the problem is with. For example, if a patient had lumbago, we choose the Spleen channel because of the day, then image it accordingly, selecting Spleen 9 as a primary point due to imaging. Additionally, we add Sp 3, the Shu Stream point and the Xi Cleft point, Sp 8, to treat the pain. Here we used a combination of holographic, imaging, chrono-acupuncture, point property and Dao Ma Zhen concepts to offer a unique solution. I haven't seen anyone else use my approach before, so therefore, I consider it unique.

JC: What are some current projects that you are working on?

RC: Well, kicking off ITARA is a big project in itself. I would like to invite speakers from other Tung lineages to come forth and do lectures, especially on the clinical use of Tung's points, especially for specific diseases. I don't believe anyone has a monopoly on the knowledge, or is the sole authority on Tung's

Acupuncture – Master Tung did not designate a robe and bowl heir. I want to stay away from practitioners who boast about how great their skill is or promote their ego, as being advanced in Chinese Medicine does not mean one is cultured or spiritually enlightened. I only want to invite go speakers who want to share and avoid the big egos and politics of some of the Tung practitioners.

I'm busy doing seminars on the basic and advanced classes monthly and have traveled to Canada, U.K. Finland, France, Spain, Australia, and throughout the U.S.A. I usually announce these at my website at http://acuchu.com.

JC: Do you provide any mentor programs for interested acupuncturists?

RC: I do provide mentorship and coaching for both new and experienced acupuncturists. Mostly it is by Socratic method in which we discuss important cases and review points, herbal formulas and clinical practices. I usually speak to my students weekly and we work on the various problems they might be experiencing, and I also pay a lot of attention to working on how they do business.

JC: Thank you.

RC: I appreciate your time in interviewing me. Thank you!

Robert Chu may be reached online at chusauli@gmail.com, by phone at (626) 487-1815, and his website is http://acuchu.com.

International Tung's Acupuncture Research Association presents:

ITARA DIPLOMATE PROGRAM

ITARA Diplomate Program is structured for Licensed Acupuncturists, and other medical professionals who want to maintain their own practices while studying. Alternatively, this program can be used as a turnkey Doctorate Acupuncture and Herbal Program to any Acupuncture School DAOM program. This program teaches in a systematic manner, the proper imparting of a complete lineage transmission from the Founder and President of ITARA, Robert Chu, PhD, L.Ac., QME.

As of recent, Master Tung's Acupuncture system has been misrepresented and only taught in a partial manner, often leading to confusion as to the proper use and context of the points. Additionally, books have come out with incorrect point locations, or simply passing down one individual's opinion of how the points should be used from their own personal perspective. Many think that Master Tung's system is only comprised of non-channel extra points, but few understand the clinical significance of the proper underlying principles and concepts. Some teach a smattering of Tung's Acupuncture, but fail to teach the proper methods of combining points, which increase their clinical efficacy.

The curriculum and content is under Robert Chu, a noted researcher and practitioner of the Tung Acupuncture system. The curriculum is designed to teach the complete core principles and concepts of

Tung's Acupuncture, including Regular and Extra points, giving the concepts to flexibly treat all diseases, and allow the practitioner to have proper access for continued research and development of this highly effective system of acupuncture.

The program will include extensive training in:

- **Tung's Regular Channel Acupuncture:** Use of the regular channel points, relationships of the channels, 5 Elements; Levels of needle insertion, use of the Antique points; Treating Symptoms; Balancing Energy; Specialized Treatment Patterns and Groupings of Points, Palm Diagnosis within the Tung System

- **Point Location and Uses:** Special Applications of the Twelve Channels, 8 Extra Channels; Yuan/Source, Lou/Connecting, Ben/Horary, Xi/Cleft, 5 element points, and Tung's 740 Extra points, learn how to coordinate Classical Acupuncture with the special set of Tung's points, along with implementation of YI Jing Acupuncture concepts

- **Traditional Diagnosis:** examining the palm/face, Diagnostic Indications; Taking Case Histories; Assessing channel imbalance; Physical Examination methods

- **Clinical Work Discussion:** Presentation of case studies, Diagnosis and Treatment of 30 submitted case studies per student

- **Treatment Planning:** Principles and Priorities; Translation of Traditional Diagnosis into Treatment Plan; Addressing the

Needs of the patient through mind, body, spirit; Methods of
Treatment; Evaluation of Treatment; Determining Future
Treatments

- **Treatment Methods:** Needling, Pricking; Moxibustion,
  Moving the Qi
- **Clinical Observation:** 12 hours arranged one on one with
  instructor

The program will be conducted entirely in English. Participants must
be prepared to devote several hours per week for individually
assigned study and practice.

Module 1: Introductory Primer Course and Points Formulary for
Pain and Internal Medicine Problems – 15 Hours

Module 2: Points on the Hands, Forearm and Upper Arm – 15
Hours Classroom, 5 hours self-study recommended

Module 3: Points on the Feet/Lower Leg/Upper Leg – 15 Hours
Classroom, 5 hours self-study recommended

Module 4: Points on the Head, Face, Ear, Ventral/Dorsal Torso –
15 Hours Classroom, 5 hours self-study recommended

Module 5: Dao Ma Zhen/Hui Ma Zhen Methods– 15 Hours
Classroom, 5 hours self-study recommended

Module 6: Difficult Cases – 15 Hours Classroom, 5 hours self-study recommended

Module 7: Master Tung Acupuncture for Female/Male Disorders– 15 Hours Classroom, 5 hours self-study recommended

Module 8: Yi Jing Acupuncture of Dr. Chen Chao – 15 Hours Classroom, 5 hours self-study recommended

Module 9: Chrono Acupuncture and Acupuncture from the Classics – 15 Hours Classroom, 5 hours self-study recommended

Module 10: Allergies and AutoImmune Disorders Module - 15 Hours Classroom, 5 hours self-study recommended

Module 11: Clinical Chinese Herbal Medicine Module - 15 Hours Classroom, 5 hours self-study recommended

Module 12: The Best of Master Tung's Acupuncture - 15 Hours Classroom, 5 hours self-study recommended

Module 13: Chinese Medicine Traumatology and Orthopedics - 15 Hours Classroom, 5 hours self-study recommended

Module 14: Prescription Refinement, and Dao of Health - 15 Hours Classroom, 5 hours self-study recommended

Module 15: Cancer Treatment Specialty, and Sports Medicine - 15 Hours Classroom, 5 hours self-study recommended

Module 16: Case Studies Presentations – 30 hours, typed and submitted

Module 16: Points Location Review Class – 15 hours

Clinic Hours: 12 hours, to be arranged

Successful course completion will earn the graduate the title:
**International Tung's Acupuncture Research Association
Diplomate of Acupuncture - Dipl. Ac. (ITARA)**

Diplomate Program in Tung's Acupuncture
Program Curriculum Hours

Seminars:

1 Introductory/Points Formulary seminar = 15 hours

14 Instructor Led material sessions = 210 hours

Practical Point Location seminar = 15 hours

Clinic = 12 hours

Subtotal = 252 hours

Independent Study, Tutorial and Research

Independent Study = 75 hours

Case Studies (4 hours x 30 cases) = 120 hours

Subtotal = 195 hours

Total Hours = 447 hours

Note: The independent study section of the course consists of intense self-study, utilizing self-study items, internalizing material covered, journaling of findings from observation hours, and practical application in the clinic. In order to maintain progress in skill development and self-development of this system of medicine, independent study projects were designed to be completed between meetings as assigned. The importance of these assignments and the time spent on them should not be underestimated. They need to be submitted on schedule for review by the instructor.

Eligibility

The program is open to licensed acupuncturists and selected students of Oriental Medicine. Admission to the program will include assessments by written application and interview. Because of the personal one-on-one attention provided to each student, class size will be limited and enrollments considered on a first come, first served basis.

The Opportunity

As the only program of its kind offered in Southern California, Tung's Acupuncture Diplomate program offers Acupuncturists the opportunity to learn this highly effective, proven Acupuncture system, noted for it's clinical efficacy, and become certified and recognized as Tung Acupuncture practitioners. The program is taught by Robert Chu, PhD, L.Ac., QME

Upon successful completion of the program, graduates will be eligible to test and receive a certificate of recognition as Diplomate in Tung's Acupuncture "Dipl.Ac. (ITARA)" issued from the International Tung's Acupuncture Research Association and be recognized for their expertise and knowledge in this system of acupuncture.

In addition, they will be eligible to participate in advanced courses, Facebook discussion groups, webpages, referrals, seminars, newsletters, conferences and clinical consultations of the International Tung's Acupuncture Research Association (ITARA).

The purpose of the Tung Acupuncture Diplomate Program is to:

- enable practitioners to provide the highest standard of care using the system of Acupuncture handed down from Tung Ching-chang
- offer a complete system, including regular channel and extra points
- standardize point location and indications
- offer the opportunity for continual growth, learning, and deeper understanding into the nature of health and well being, freely sharing information amongst members prepare and train a new generation of practitioners who will carry on this tradition and system

BIBLIOGRAPHY

Master Tung's Acupuncture Primer by Robert Chu, PhD, L.Ac., QME, Self-published

Master Tung's Upper Limb Acupuncture by Robert Chu, PhD, L.Ac., QME, Self-published

Master Tung's Lower Limb Acupuncture by Robert Chu, PhD, L.Ac., QME, Self-published

Master Tung's Head and Torso Acupuncture by Robert Chu, PhD, L.Ac., QME, Self-published

Introduction to Tung's Acupuncture by Dr. Chuan-Min Wang, Published 2013, Chinese Tung Acupuncture Institute Publications, ISBN 978-1-4675-2684-5

Acupuncturist's Handbook Revised Edition by Kuen Shii Tsay, Published: 1996, ISBN: 0-9647445-0-3

Chinese Acupuncture and Moxibustion by Xin-nong Cheng, Published: 1996, ISBN: 7-119-01758-6

Five Elements and Ten Stems by Kiiko Matsumoto, Stephen Birch, Published: 1983, ISBN: 0-912111-25-9

Fundamentals of Chinese Acupuncture, by Andrew Ellis, Nigel Wiseman, Published: 1991, ISBN: 0-912111-33-X

Grasping the Wind, the Meaning of Chinese Acupuncture Points by Andrew Ellis, Nigel Wiseman, Published: 1989, ISBN: 0-912111-19-4

Insights of a Senior Acupuncturist by Miriam Lee, Published: 1992
ISBN: 0-936185-33-3

Manual of Acupuncture by Peter Deadman, Mazin Al-Khafaji, Published: 1998, ISBN: 0-9510546-7-8

Optimum Time for Acupuncture, by Liu Bing Quan, Published: 1988, ISBN: 7-5331-0282-7

Practical Application of Meridian Style Acupuncture by John Pirog, Published: 1996, ISBN: 1-881896-13-7

Sticking to the Point Vol 1 by Bob Flaws, Published: 1998, ISBN: 0-936185-17-1

Sticking to the Point Vol 2 by Bob Flaws, Published: 1998, ISBN: 0-936185-97-X

Study of Daoist Acupuncture by Liu Zheng-Cai, Published: 1999, ISBN: 1-891945-08-X

Fundamentals of Chinese Medicine (PAPER) by Nigel Wiseman, Andrew Ellis, Published: 1996, ISBN: 0-912111-44-5

Clinical Applications Yellow Emperors Canon by Hong Tu Wang, Published: 1999, ISBN: 7-80005-444-6

Practice of Chinese Medicine by Giovanni Maciocia, Published: 1994, ISBN: 0-443-04305-1

Classic of Difficulties (Nan Jing Translation) by Bob Flaws, Published 1999, ISBN: 1-891845-07-1

Early Chinese Medical Literature by Donald Harper, Published: 1998, ISBN: 0-7103-0582-6

Huang Di Nei Jing Su Wen by Paul Unschuld, Published: 2003, ISBN: 0-520-23322-0

Ling Shu, The Spiritual Pivot by Jing-Nuan Wu, 1993, ISBN: 0-8248-2631-0

Master Hua's Classic of the Central Viscera by Hua Tuo, 1999, ISBN: 0-936185-43-0

Master Tong's Acupuncture by Miriam Lee, 1992, ISBN: 0-936185-37-6

Medicine in China: Nan-Ching, Classic of Difficult Issues by Paul Unschuld, 1986, ISBN: 0-520-05372-9

A Complete Translation of The Yellow Emperor's Classics of Internal Medicine and the Difficult Classic – Henry Lu Translation, Published by the **International College of Traditional Chinese Medicine**, Vancouver, Canada.

Medical Classic of the Yellow Emperor (ILLUSTRATED) by Ming Zhu, 2001, ISBN: 7-119-02664-X

Yellow Emperor's Canon Internal Medicine by Wang Bing, Nelson Liansheng Wu, 1999, ISBN: 7-5046-2231-1

Yellow Emperor's Classic of Medicine by Maoshing Ni, 1995, ISBN: 1-57062-080-6

Yellow Emperor's Classic of Internal Medicine by Ilza Veith, 1949, ISBN: 0-520-22936-3

Statements of Fact in Traditional Chinese Medicine, Completely Revised & Expanded by Bob Flaws, 1994, ISBN: 0-936185-52-X

Tung's Orthodox Acupuncture, by Palden Carson, MD, Hsin Ya Publications, Ltd, 1988

Tung's Acupuncture, by Palden Carson, MD, Hsin Ya Publications, Ltd, 1973

Personal notes from lectures by Dr. Young, Robert Chu 2001-2005

Personal notes from Dr. Tan's lectures, Robert Chu, 2001-2004.

Sources In Chinese:

董氏针灸注疏, 2011-03, 刘毅

Ci Xue Liao Fa, by Wang Xiu Zhen, Zhi Yuan Publishing, Taiwan 1990

Dong Si Qi Xue Zhen Jiu Xue, by Young Wei-Chieh, Zhi Yuan Publishing, Taiwan 1992

Dong Si Qi Xue Zhen Jiu Xue, by Young Wei-Chieh, Zhong Yi Gu Jing Publishing, China 1994

Zhong Hua Shi Deng Zhen Liao Fa, by Liu Yan, Shang Hai Ke Xue Publishing, China 1992

Zhong Hua Ji He Xue, by Liu Yan, Shang Hai Ke Xue Publishing, China 2002

Zhong Hua Qi Xue Da Cheng, by Liu Yan, Shang Hai Ke Xue Publishing, China 2002, ISBN 7-5439-1738-6/R 444

Zhen Jiu Jing Wei, by Young Wei-Chieh, Zhi Yuan Publishing, Taiwan 1985, ISBN: 957-8609-43-4

Zhen Jiu Wu Shu Xue Ying Yong, by Young Wei-Chieh, Zhi Yuan Publishing, Taiwan 1981

Zhen Jiu Ban Xue Xue, by Young Wei-Chieh, Zhi Yuan Publishing, Taiwan 1980

Taiwan Dong Si Zhen Jiu Jing Xue Xue, by Li Guo Zhen, Zhi Yuan Publishing, Taiwan 1994

Taiwan Dong Si Ji Chu Jiang Yi, by Li Guo Zhen, Zhi Yuan Publishing, Taiwan 1995

Taiwan Dong Si Zhen Jiu Zhen Duan Xue, by Li Guo Zhen, Zhi Yuan Publishing, Taiwan 1994

Taiwan Dong Si Zhen Jiu Jing Xue Xue, by Li Guo Zhen, Zhi Yuan Publishing, Taiwan 1994

Taiwan Dong Si Zhen Jiu Dao Ma Zhen Ci Liao Fa, by Li Guo Zhen, Zhi Yuan Publishing, Taiwan 1994

Taiwan Dong Si Zhen Jiu Shou Zhen Liao Fa, by Li Guo Zhen, Zhi Yuan Publishing, Taiwan 1996

Dong Si Zhen Jiu Fang Xue Liao Fa, by Li Guo Zhen, Zhi Yuan Publishing, Taiwan 1993

Taiwan Dong Si Zhen Jiu Shou Jiao Dui Ying Zhen Fa, by Li Guo Zhen, Zhi Yuan Publishing, Taiwan 1996

Taiwan Dong Si Qi Xue Fu Ke Zhen Ci Liao Fa, by Li Guo Zhen, Zhi Yuan Publishing, Taiwan 1996

Taiwan Dong Si Jiao Yuan Jing Bing Zhen Ci Liao Fa, by Li Guo Zhen, Zhi Yuan Publishing, Taiwan 1996

Dong Si Zhen Jiu Tu Pu Jing Duan Shang/Xia Pian, by Hu Bing Quan, Zhi Yuan Publishing, Taiwan 1998

Dong Si Qi Xue Tu Pu Zhi Liao Fa, by Hu Bing Quan, Zhi Yuan Publishing, Taiwan 1988

Dong Si Zhen Jiu Qi Xue Jing Nian Lu, by Lai Jin Hong, Zhi Yuan Publishing, Taiwan 1987

About the Author:

Robert Chu (Chu Sau Lei) began the study of the Chinese martial and healing arts since childhood. Robert is a California Licensed Acupuncturist and Herbalist in Pasadena, CA. He specializes in the Master Tung and Optimal Acupuncture methods of painless Acupuncture where he effectively treats pain, industrial medicine, sports injuries, and neuromusculoskeletal disorders. He also treats a wide variety of internal diseases, gynecological disorders, and side-effects from cancer treatments. He is appointed by the **Industrial Medical Council** as a **Qualified Medical Evaluator (QME).**

Dr. Chu was formerly affiliated with the **St. Vincent Medical Center, Center for Health and Healing**, as the first fulltime Acupuncturist on staff and treated cancer patients with Acupuncture, Herbal Therapy Qigong and Tai Chi. Robert is a former faculty member of **Samra University of Oriental Medicine** in Los Angeles, where he taught acupuncture. He graduated from Samra University with a Master of Science in Oriental Medicine. Not satisfied with his education, he went on to study with the renowned **Young Wei-chieh**, student of Master Tung; and **Chen Chao**, creator of I Ching Acupuncture. His studies in classical acupuncture led him to create the system that he calls "Optimal Acupuncture".

Dr. Chu has also taught Tai Chi and Qigong at Loyola Law School. He volunteers regularly at Pasadena's Wellness Community, where he does monthly lectures on Acupuncture and Herbal Therapy for Cancer Patients and a weekly lifestyle/nutrition and Qi Gong class for cancer patients.   In July of 2004, he was the Acupuncturist to Olympic Athletes in Sacramento, CA at the Olympic Trials.

Robert also lectures nationally and internationally on Acupuncture and Chinese Medicine to provide continuing education to MD's and Acupuncturists. He has spread his version of the Master Tung's Acupuncture throughout his organization called ITARA (International Tung's Acupuncture Research Association) with branches in the U.K., Canada, Finland, Spain, France, Australia, and throughout the United States. He has lectured at Emperor's College of TCM, CSOMA, Five Branches, University of East West Medicine, American College of Acupuncture and Oriental Medicine, Acupuncture Integrative Medicine College, NESA, the American Cancer Society and other functions as a dynamic and entertaining speaker.

In the martial arts world, he specializes in combat application and health aspects with a focus on the *Yip Man Wing Chun Kuen* system as taught by Hawkins Cheung, the *Yuen Kay-San* and *Gulao Wing Chun Kuen* systems as taught by Kwan Jong-Yuen, and the Yik Kam Wing Chun system as taught by Hendrik Santo. He is the co-author of **Complete Wing Chun**, (Charles E. Tuttle Co., Inc, 1998), author of **The Essence of Wing Chun** (3 volumes, 2004) and has written many articles for *Inside Kung Fu*, *Martial Arts Legends*, *Inside Martial Arts*, *Martial Arts Combat Sports* and other publications.

Dr. Chu was featured in the book, ***Kung Fu Masters* (CFW Enterprises),** in 2002, and **Wing Chun Masters** in 2013. Robert Chu has been formally involved in the martial arts since 1972, specializing in *wing chun kuen* and its weapons. Having learned Yip Man wing chun kuen from several prominent instructors such as his current teacher, Hawkins Cheung, and the Yuen Kay-San and Gulao systems from his good friend and teacher Kwan Jong-Yuen, as well as the Yik Kam Wing Chun system as taught by Hendrik Santo, he has also researched several other branches of the system. In addition, he has a background in the empty hand fist and weapons sets of Hung ga kuen under Yee Chi Wai, and the Lama martial arts as taught by Chen Tai Shan. He is one of the last disciples and a successor to Lui Yon-Sang's flying dragon tiger gate combat pole in the United States.

Robert can be reached at: (626) 345-0441   chusauli@gmail.com 1028 N. Lake Avenue, Suite 107, Pasadena, CA 91104 or for more information on the internet, please see:

http://acuchu.com

http://www.acupuncturetoday.com/archives2003/jan/01carter.html

Dr. Chu will be available for further seminars. Please feel free to contact him with the information above.

Appendix:

Using the points mentioned in this manual to treat a few common ailments:

Neck Pain
1) St 41
2) San Chong Hui Ma Set
3) Qi Hu

Shoulder Pain
1) Shen Guan or Tian Huang, palpate for ashi reaction
2) Ce San Li, Ce Xia San Li
3) San Chong Hui Ma Set
4) Qi Hu

Knee Pain
1) Lu 5, LI 11
2) Huo Ying, Huo Zhu

Back Pain
1) Ling Gu, Da Bai, UB 40
2) San Jiu Li

Sciatica
1) Ling Gu, Da Bai, GB 34
2) San Jiu Li

Toe Pain
1) Zu Wu Hu 3

Heel Pain
1) Zu Wu Hu 5

Conjunctivitis
1) Huo Ying, Huo Zhu

Otitis Media
1) Ce San Li, Ce Xia San Li

Toothache
1) Men Jin

Sinusitis
1) Si Ma San Hui Ma Set
2) Men Jin

Dysmenorrhea
1) Fu Ke, Xia San Huang, Huo Ying, Huo Zhu

Fibromyalgia
1) Xia San Huang, Huo Ying, Huo Zhu, San Chong

Chronic Fatigue
1) Xia San Huang, San Chong, Huo Ying, Huo Zhu

Hangover
1) Bi Yi, Huo Ying, Huo Zhu

Index:

For a detailed treatment formulary on treating Pain and Internal Medicine disorders, please refer to my <u>Master Tung's Acupuncture for Pain</u> and my <u>Master Tung's Acupuncture for Internal Medicine Disorders</u>. For those wishing to expand their repertoire of points and learn how to create their own acupuncture point prescriptions using Master Tung's Acupuncture would best to refer to my <u>The Best of Master Tung's Acupuncture</u>.

Qi Hu 七 虎 – Seven Tigers - 127

Ren Huang 人皇 – Human Emperor – 129

San Chong 三重 – Third Layer - 128
Shen Guan 腎關, also known as Tian Huang Fu 天皇附 – Kidney
Gate, Heaven Emperor Appendage - 129
Si Ma Zhong 駟馬中 – Chariot Center - 133
Si Ma Shang 駟馬上 – Chariot Upper - 133
Si Ma Xia 駟馬下 – Chariot Lower – 133

Tian Huang 天 皇 – Heaven Emperor - 129

Wai San Guan 外 三 關 – External Three Gates - 106
Wu Hu 五虎 – Five Tigers - 119

Xia Jiu Li 下九里 – Lower Nine Miles - 134

Yi Chong 一 重 – First Layer - 128

Zhong Jiu Li 中九里 – Center Nine Miles - 134
Zu Wu Hu 足五虎 / Foot Five Tigers - 123

www.ingramcontent.com/pod-product-compliance
Lightning Source LLC
Chambersburg PA
CBHW051911170526
45168CB00001B/335